T0260281

Off the Hook

First published in 1985, *Off the Hook* describes all the signs and symptoms of drug addiction, alcoholism or compulsive gambling in teenagers, but more importantly suggests constructive ways parents can help. Teenage disorder, and especially addiction, can cause serious family damage. Fear, guilt and shame can paralyse effective action and even make matters worse. Helen Bethune, drawing on research among recovered addicts, troubled teenagers and suffering families, throws new light on this problem. There is hope, and there are positive steps which parents can take to help their children towards recovery. This book is highly informative and essential reading not only for the afflicted but for all parents fearful of the prevalence of drugs among youngsters today, and for teachers and social workers at every level.

Off the Hook

Coping with Addiction

Helen Bethune

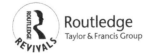

Routledge
Taylor & Francis Group

First published in 1985
By Methuen

This edition first published in 2022 by Routledge
4 Park Square, Milton Park, Abingdon, Oxon, OX14 4RN
and by Routledge
605 Third Avenue, New York, NY 10017

Routledge is an imprint of the Taylor & Francis Group, an informa business

© 1985 by Helen Bethune

Publisher's Note
The publisher has gone to great lengths to ensure the quality of this reprint but points out that some imperfections in the original copies may be apparent.

Disclaimer
The publisher has made every effort to trace copyright holders and welcomes correspondence from those they have been unable to contact.

ISBN: 978-1-032-42614-3 (hbk)
ISBN: 978-1-003-36351-4 (ebk)
ISBN: 978-1-032-42617-4 (pbk)

Book DOI 10.4324/9781003363514

HELEN BETHUNE

OFF THE HOOK

Coping With Addiction

Methuen · London

First published in Great Britain
by Methuen Children's Books Ltd
11 New Fetter Lane, London EC4P 4EE
Copyright © 1985 by Helen Bethune
Line drawings by Kevin Ryan copyright© 1985
by Methuen Children's Books Ltd

Printed in Great Britain

British Library Cataloguing in Publication Data

Bethune, Helen
　　Off the hook: coping with addiction.
　　1. Drug abuse
　　I. Title
　　362.2193　　　　　RC564

ISBN 0-416-53280-2
ISBN 0-416-53300-0 Pbk

CONTENTS

Illustrations

All the people in this book exist. Of course names and descriptions have been changed so you cannot recognise them. However it is quite possible that you may recognise *yourself* in some of the characters or some of the situations.

H.B.

addict n. one who is dependent on, finds it impossible to give up, a habit, vice etc., e.g. drug-taking
addicted adj. enslaved to, dependent on
addiction n.
addictive adj. inclined to cause dependence

From Chambers Pocket
20th Century Dictionary (1984)

ONE

TROUBLESOME TEENAGERS

It is the nature of teenagers to misbehave. If they don't then perhaps a parent has something to worry about. But there are degrees of misbehaviour. It is one thing for a youngster to refuse to do the washing up. It is quite another to take a fix of heroin in your bathroom.

Paradoxically, the treatment for both may be identical. And the treatment begins with you – the parents.

Let's get a few basic facts out of the way first. It's extremely difficult being a parent in the seventies and eighties. There are no precedents in living memory for what parents are facing today. At the turn of the century there was a drink and drug problem. In the thirties there was massive unemployment. Today we have both of these and an extended school leaving age, which chains teenagers to school and home till they are past sixteen. Until the legal age of marriage, in fact.

Yet, when everything else is crumbling, when the education system has failed to persuade thousands of young pupils to go willingly to school, when the makers and enforcers of law have failed to stop traffic in drugs, when jobs do not exist even for those with the coveted piece of paper, there are always parents to fall back on. Parents are there to pick up the tab and to take the blame. Let us be clear about this; most parents love their children dearly and want the very best for them. If you didn't love your child you wouldn't be reading this book now. As parents we are often mistaken, often get it wrong, but we do try to do our best for our offspring.

Parents are also subjected to an appalling amount of garbage from 'experts' – which is very often social engineering under another mask. During the last war, women's labour was required in the forces, the factories and the fields. Miraculously crèches and nurseries sprang up all over Britain and nobody mentioned deprived children. But when the men came back and needed jobs, suddenly a rash of 'experts' announced in tones of doom that any mother who left her child to go to work was likely to spawn a delinquent. 'Maternal deprivation' was the cry. Crèches and nurseries began closing with unseemly speed.

The aftermath of this barrage lingers on today, despite subsequent evidence that quality – not quantity – is the most important part of mothering. An hour's *good* mothering a day is enough. One marriage in every three ends in divorce. Single mothers, wives of the poor and the unemployed often must work if the family is to eat. Yet working mothers are still singled out for blame when the going gets tough, when the kids become troublesome. The professionals and experts conveniently forget all the other children of working mothers who do not disturb society's tranquillity.

Yet troublesome teenagers – whether they are defined as difficult, delinquent or drug-addicted – can be found in every section of society. In magistrates' courts, detention centres, probation offices and drug units, you can see youngsters from every sort of home, from every class, colour, creed and family unit, whether the parents are single, paired, happy or hating, in law or in common law, with brothers and sisters or as only children.

The deepest influence on parents comes from their own experience of having had parents. We've all been parented, sometimes well, sometimes badly, mostly a bit of both. When we come to be parents ourselves we often do a great many things, almost instinctively, in the same way that our parents did. Old records, playing in the head, from oft-repeated warnings and injunctions by our mothers and fathers, impel us to do a lot of things apparently automatically. In other ways it is hard not to overcompensate for some perceived mistake of our own parents. Don't we all know people who push their children into having or doing things they themselves were denied – whether the children want it or not? Haven't we done this ourselves? Whether we behave in the same way as our parents, or use them as awful warnings and do the opposite, the way we were brought up conditions the way we behave as parents ourselves.

Today there are many issues that simply did not arise for most of our own parents.

For teenagers, the world, new-minted, shows itself in black and white. So let's face the big one first. When we were children, the world was still a safe place – with a future. We have grown up and lived to see our children become teenagers. But for them? Whatever your view of the nuclear debate, the Bomb (in vast quantity) exists. Whether by design or by error, the elimination of the world is on the cards. The unthinkable has become the possible. While you and I may choose to look the other way, this option is not open to a great many teenagers. Shades of grey painted out in SALT talks, in peace initiatives, in deterrence and in political commentaries do not rub away the stark fact that many sensitive teenagers do not expect to see their own children become teenagers. According to the forty six eminent scientists who record these things, the clock of lethal destruction stands at three minutes to midnight. Most teen-agers are quite aware of this.

Our own parents gave us no answers to the question: 'Why should I bother when the Bomb could go off any time?' – for the good reason that even 20 years ago there was very little likeli-hood of this happening. Nobody needed to ask the question.

The next issue – almost as big – which parents now are forced to confront, is, 'What's the point when the planet is going to be finished in fifty years anyway?' Our own parents did not have to consider the rape of rain forests, pollution and acid rain in the First and Second Worlds, megadeath through starvation and pillage of agricultural land in the Third World. How do we answer these questions in the context of helping with the washing up or using a bit of cannabis now and again? Nobody has given us any answers because nobody asked the question before.

Exams, qualifications, employment prospects and sex have all been batted around between parents and young people since recorded memory. Every parent has a view on these things and it is either a carbon copy from their own parents, a mirror image

3

of it, or a thoughtful, up-dated compromise. These are not new questions.

But in the last fifteen or twenty years there has developed a great credibility gap. All the major institutions of the country are seen to be crumbling. No longer do adults stick together to defend 'right' and condemn 'wrong' with the same surefootedness they did when we were young.

Early in the sixties, there was a small court case. It involved a young girl who went to school in bright, fluorescent socks. The headmaster sent her home because she was not wearing proper uniform. Her father sent her back to school the next day, again wearing the socks. The girl was sent home again – and so it went on, until the father took the headmaster to court, on the grounds that the headmaster was denying the child her right to education. The judge decided in favour of the father. At the time this appeared to be a landmark. Previously – even a few years earlier – it would have been unthinkable for a parent not to accept the view of the school. 'Authority' presented a united face. Parents, teachers, the police, the courts, the law, government, the church all stood together, safe in their certainties.

What is 'right' and what is 'wrong' has grown increasingly hard to define, particularly when it comes to institutions. Nobody in reach of the media today can be in any doubt that government, politicians, the police, the judiciary, the education system, the churches, the city, the trades unions and even the charities often have feet of clay – or worse. The media expose them relentlessly. For young people there can be no institutional heroes or heroines ... with the exception of some of the still sacred Royal Family. However as a model for action this is hardly useful. Royalty happens by birth or by marriage, so the possibilities of following in that route are somewhat restricted.

Perhaps the last institutional hero that young people could look up to was John F. Kennedy. Yet he was hardly in his grave when the muck began being raked. Probably the only public figure in the last century to have emerged with his integrity intact is Einstein – though if he'd accepted the Presidency of Israel and become really 'institutionalised', almost certainly someone somewhere would have produced a book, a series in the press, or a TV documentary entitled 'EINSTEIN – THE DARK TRUTH' – even if it had to be invented.

Conscientious parents today have to think through a great many issues both large and small which our own parents took for granted. Drugs are something which our parents most certainly did not have to cope with. Here and there, in a few sections of society, heroin and cocaine have always been around. And alcohol, of course, everywhere. But the explosion of illicit and unexpected drugs which has now hit almost every part of the country, is something quite different from anything our parents encountered. Almost every child over twelve has been offered – or used – an illegal drug ... or knows people who use them. How many parents today could have said the same at the age of twelve?

No parent in this decade can safely ignore the possibility that their young child may be using or abusing drugs. Or they may be gambling compulsively. Either way these activities don't always show at first. What is more, questioning is not likely to get you very far. If pressed hard enough many will admit to using a bit of cannabis now and then – with the justification that it is 'less addictive than alcohol'. This lets them off the hook and can lull your own suspicions for some time.

It is only behaviour that tells the truth. *Their* behaviour – together with *your* reactions to it.

Behaviour and Misbehaviour

I use the word behaviour because that's where the action is. Motivations, attitudes, emotions and intentions are all invisible. All these are expressed in *behaviour*. It is behaviour we live with.

Living with teenagers is rarely undiluted joy. Their mental, physical and emotional growth occurs in spurts. Since it is important for their development that they shake off parental dependency they usually become secretive. They also become defiant, argumentative or (the other side of the coin) sullen and uncommunicative. On the outside this may look like lack of love. Of course, it is nothing of the kind. When these bids for

5

independence are expressed merely in general untidiness, lack of cooperation and lengthy, semi-secret telephone calls, a parent may well live through it, however tiresome.

But, and this is the big 'but', there's a different kind of misbehaviour. The difference cannot be defined in an exact way, because every home is different. What is permissible in one family may be totally beyond the pale in another. Only *you* know – for only you live with it. What is more, your children know, because they have lived with you all their lives. There is a point beyond which misbehaviour becomes unacceptable behaviour. In your gut you know when that boundary has been passed.

Probably you know because you are in deep despair. You are worn out with worry, with pleading and begging. You are exhausted with rows and possibly frightened by violence. You are angry and hurt that your beloved child appears to be turning into a monster. They may be stealing from you or demanding money with menaces. You fear for their sanity, or your own. You are probably getting tranquillizers or sleeping pills from your doctor. You feel you are a failure – that you've done it all wrong. You are consumed with guilt and shame. You are full of envy of parents who don't have your problems and with self-pity that this should happen to you. You may even, if you know they are using drugs, fear for their very lives. You are confused and desolate and you feel you have nowhere to turn. Your family is alone in its misery.

Help Outside the Home?

Asking for help is terribly difficult for most parents with a deeply troubled child. Usually the GP is the first person a parent turns to, especially mothers. And usually the GP offers tranquillizers. This is about as useful as giving someone ointment for a headache. It may, for a day or two, make it slightly easier to drift through the day, but it will not solve the problem and it might even turn her into a compulsive pill-popper herself.

Other relatives may be sympathetic, but quite often give very bad advice. They may even depress you further by digging out dreadful family skeletons who came to a sticky end. Doting grannies and grandfathers may simply deny there is a problem. 'Kids will be kids – they'll grow out of it.'

Friends, notably friends with children who don't seem to be difficult, are even worse. A distressed parent, hoping for a magic formula, may tell a 'successful' friend some of the story, (rarely the whole truth – it is too shaming) and be met with either incomprehension or dismay. Unless you talk to someone who really understands the problem, then you feel you're at the receiving end of either contempt or pity. This is bad for you and won't solve anything.

On the other hand, the parents of your son or daughter's friends, who are themselves suffering exactly the way you are, are unlikely to be helpful either. Both sets of parents probably blame the others' child for leading their own offspring astray.

One distressed single parent had a very troubled, verbally violent and sometimes physically threatening son of seventeen, using cannabis, alcohol, LSD, magic mushrooms and assorted other substances (as he later was to tell her). She tried the following agencies:

1. Her doctor, who prescribed pills for her.
2. A psychiatrist, who saw them both and told her she was a dominant mother, that her son was merely acting out her own 'penis envy'.
3. The Social Services. They agreed to write and ask her son if he'd care to see them. The letter came six weeks later. He ignored it.
4. The Probation Service. She was told that unless she could provide the police with evidence of physical damage to herself or her home, they could do nothing.
5. A lawyer. The advice was that she had to keep the youth since he was too old to be put into care. Although he was not attending school regularly, he was technically still being educated – and the boy's claim that she *had* to keep him was correct, in law.

'It's Just A Phase'

Possibly the most unhelpful thing which can be said to a suffering parent who asks for help about a troubled teenager is the dreaded phrase, 'It's just a phase, they'll grow out of it.'

It may in fact be true … but it doesn't do a thing to help you right now. Right now you're living in the middle of confusion, fear, lies, anger, disturbance, disorder and heaven knows what else. Right now, you need to know what to DO, because it is all happening around you. The fact that they may grow out of it in some unforseeable future isn't a lot of help.

Also, your fears may not be groundless, in the sense that certain people are very definitely at risk. Drug addiction, alcoholism and compulsive gambling are all likely to lead to death, to prison – or both. Anorexia can be fatal. Drug addiction and alcoholism may lead to permanent mental impairment. Why some people become addicted while others do not is not clear, even to the many scientists, doctors and psychiatrists who are constantly researching the field.

However, the symptoms of teenage disorder (which *may* be grown out of) are usually similar, if not identical to the symptoms of the addict. It is better to be safe than sorry. Addiction is no respecter of persons. It stiketh where it listeth.

In the teeth of the experts' uncertainties, but at the receiving end of all the blame, is it any wonder that loving parents feel hopeless, desperate and inadequate? Parental breakdown – and even suicide are not by any means unknown.

Parent-Power

You will perhaps be surprised to find me now talking as it were, out of two sides of my mouth at once. I am now going to tell you something of the utmost importance. It is that for all our warts and imperfections, for all our mistakes and errors, parents wield an enormous amount of clout. We may not be God – but we have one hell of a lot of power.

For several decades, parent-power has only been seen in its

negative aspect. Since Freud turned his jaundiced eyes on parents (and particularly mothers) as the source and supply of most mental disorder, much psychological and psychiatric tradition has tended to trace all trouble back to parents.

The unintended consequence of this has been that parents, just by *being* parents, feel themselves always likely to be in the wrong. Whatever they do, they get clobbered. They're too permissive or too strict, too demanding or not demanding enough. Bombarded by experts and professionals, attacked by the helping professions, put down by educators, social workers, do-gooders and many politicians, they are at a loss what to do for the best. Parent-power has come to be seen only as a force for destruction. Rubbish. Parent-power can be positive and healing as none other. You have parent-power. It is there for you to recover. It was born in you the day your child was born. This book is about helping you to recognise and realise your own parent-power so that you may learn to use it to help and heal both yourself and your troubled child.

You are not inadequate. Like vast numbers of bewildered parents you have simply been numbed by events and social pressures into fear of getting it wrong. Now we're going to start getting it right.

If the behaviour of your teenager is causing you concern, you can wait till the cows come home for action from society that is really effective. For years truant officers, educators, politicians, police, probation officers, customs officers, well-meaning professionals and voluntary bodies have tried to get young people to behave 'properly'. But the misery goes on – behind lace curtains and trendy blinds, behind castle walls and in council houses. To judge from the figures of truancy, juvenile crime, under-age drunkenness, drugs-related offences and general delinquency, the experts aren't having a lot of success, are they?

Because there are no longer any agreed rules about many issues, because there are no longer heroes and heroines in the same way as there used to be, the one constant in anyone's life is their family. How our mother and father behave and perceive us, affects everyone. Deep down inside everyone is a desire for parental approval and love. It may be heavily disguised, even hotly denied, but it's there. If you really think deeply about yourself, isn't it true? Don't you really want to be the kind of person your own parents would be proud of, in every part of your life?

Teenagers – however badly they may behave – are no different. They may be better at disguising it, but underneath, there's a deep desire to be the kind of person *you* would be proud of. Trouble is, the lines of communication have probably got so twisted, neither of you is making sense to the other. Comment becomes criticism, discussion becomes argument, concern is interpreted as overprotection, independence is seen as disobedience ... and so on.

Somehow it is necessary to break through. Since someone has to do something about the situation, that someone is going to have to be YOU. It's you who will have to change – to start making constructive use of your parent-power. What's more, you and you alone can compete and *win* against all the other forces in the outside world beyond the family.

What is Addiction Anyway?

There are many definitions of addiction or, as it is sometimes called, dependence, and numerous theories about it are batted about by scientists, doctors, psychiatrists and other pundits. I am not about to go into these. I want to discuss addiction as it actually affects the family.

People can get all kinds of addictions – not just drink, drugs, nicotine, gambling and food – they can also get addicted to work, to money and to a dozen other things. Many addictions can be damaging. One father of my acquaintance lost two wives and four children because of his obsessional devotion to his career at the expense of his family. But this addiction will not land him in either a psychiatric institution or prison though it may shorten his life. In simple terms, the addictions we are concerned with here are those which not only shorten life, but also lead inexorably to either a penal or a psychiatric institution. I shall therefore not discuss the perils of nicotine, work, money and the rest. Food falls somewhere in between. The behaviour of some types of anorexics parallels that of addicts, but our main concern will be with alcohol, drugs and gambling.

It is generally held that there are two types of addiction – physical and psychological. People are said to be physically addicted when:

a: they experience physical craving for the object of the addiction, and
b: they show physical symptoms of discomfort when the object of their addiction is withdrawn.

The most dramatic is the epileptic fit suffered by an alcoholic when suddenly deprived of alcohol. This can cause death in certain circumstances. Therefore doctors, drying-out clinics, and treatment centres sometimes prescribe a stabilizing drug when alcohol use is stopped.

The physical symptoms of heroin withdrawal are painful but neither protracted nor lethal. 'A bad dose of 'flu' for about five days is how it is described by people who have gone through it. People do not die from sudden withdrawal of heroin. The horrors of cold turkey are not entirely a myth – but they are certainly exaggerated by addicts themselves and by dealers. They are considerably less than the horrors that await the addict who goes on using.

Sudden withdrawal from heavy use of amphetamines (speed) is, however, extremely dangerous. Shortly after the drug is stopped, serious amphetamine psychosis will strike the user. This is a severe breakdown involving hallucinations, delusions or (often) violent behaviour. The patient may require straight-jacket treatment before sedation can be given. Serious psychological damage may follow for months, years or even life.

If a heavy valium user suddenly stops rather than tapers off, he or she will almost certainly suffer from disorientation, hallucinations and other psychiatric disturbances in varying degrees.

All right. We now know a bit about physical withdrawal from some addictions – but we all know people who've been dried out, or come off or given it up or gone on the wagon – and sooner or later returned to their habit. This is where we come up against the mysterious force of psychological addiction – what is sometimes referred to as the 'mental obsession'. For psychological addiction acts like a magnet to draw the addict time and time again back to the path of self-destruction.

There are many who believe that addiction is intrinsic in certain personalities. How otherwise can we explain the fact that a great many people can drink alcohol even in considerable quantities without falling into the pit of alcoholism? How can it be that some people can, without discomfort, come off almost any kind of drug or stop gambling after years of heavy betting? Unfortunately, there are no clear pointers to the particular personality types at special risk. Also there is no doubt that heavy usage of alcohol or drugs or excessive gambling is liable to lead to addiction. It is a different, longer road, but the end is usually the same: an unlovely death, or a stay in an institution.

An interesting fact which concerns these three addictions is their frequent interchangeability. One counsellor has been heard to say: 'You can always tell an addict. If they cannot get the drug they love, they'll love the drug they can get.' For this reason, many former drug users either immediately or later turn to excessive use of alcohol. Alcoholics, off the booze, sometimes start heavy gambling. Gamblers may start drinking. Very often it is a three-way permutation.

What Causes Addiction?

A lot of people have advanced theories – but the facts unfortunately do not accommodate themselves easily. Addiction cannot be put down to unhappy homes, to social conditions, to overwork, to lack of work, to deprived childhoods, to being an only child, to coming from a large family, to being rich, to being poor, to being famous or infamous. The fact is that addicts come from all backgrounds and all life-styles. What they have in common are symptoms which appear when addiction is happening. For this (and other reasons) addiction is known as an illness – and indeed alcoholism is accepted by the World Health Organisation as such – one of the three biggest killer

12

diseases in the world – up there with cancer and heart disease.

Addiction certainly is not a moral weakness – though sick addicts will usually lose their personal moral values. This too is a symptom of the illness, and exceedingly difficult for the family to live with – or even to understand.

In some respects addiction resembles diabetes in that it can grow slowly and insidiously, or can strike quite suddenly and unexpectedly, often after a shock. Brenda, aged forty four, had hardly drunk alcohol in her life, just the odd glass of sherry at Christmas and birthdays. She lived contentedly with her husband and seventeen year old daughter in a neat suburban house. Every Friday she used to meet her husband for a meal and a visit to the cinema. One Friday he did not turn up. She waited for about an hour, and, filled with foreboding, finally went home. An hour later two policewomen came to the door. They told her that her husband had had a heart attack and died suddenly in the street. They sat in her sitting room and the police women tried to comfort her. One of them said, 'Can I make you a cup of tea dear?' She found herself saying, 'My husband keeps some scotch in that cupboard'. So the police-woman gave her a scotch. She was later to say she didn't put the bottle down for three years except during two brief periods when she was hospitalised and dried out.

Some teenagers are hooked mercilessly from their first drink, pill, fix or bet. They might not like the taste of the drug – but they crave for what it does to them. They may be sick, suffer agonies, loss of money, face or friends, but the drug – whether it's speed, beer or a fruit machine – is more powerful than the person. Others get hooked more slowly. Some don't get hooked at all.

There is one big drawback to to all this. All three groups will *say* they are not addicted. The first two lie (the instant addict and the slow-burn addict) – because at the beginning they don't even know it themselves. Later they deny *because* of the addiction.

How are you to know into which group your youngster falls? The answer is, you don't. Not at the beginning, at any rate.

13

Addiction is a Treatable Illness

Alcoholics are treatable patients. Thus says the American Medical Association.

So are drug addicts and compulsive gamblers.

There *is* hope. If you walk down any street in any town or city you will encounter many recovered alcoholics, addicts and former gamblers. They will look just like you and me. But they are well, straight and sober today. If you have reason to believe that your son or daughter is on the way to addiction, the first thing to keep telling yourself, however hard it may be, is that your child is suffering from an illness. They are not subjects for blame – and neither are you. We'll talk more about guilt and self-blame later.

The second thing to remember is that he or she is treatable. They can recover. There really is hope. Every one of the people you will read about in this book have recovered, or are parents whose youngsters have recovered from one or other of these addictions. And there are hundreds of thousands more.

The third thing is to use your common sense. You want treatment for your child? Think about it like any other commodity you are in need of. If a crazy driver crashed into your car and you needed a good repair garage, you would hardly be likely to take the advice of the lunatic driver, would you? You'd ask someone who'd had a good repair job done. Until your troubled child is well, it is recommended that you take little notice of their suggestions for treatment. It is no secret that certain members of the medical profession especially in Harley Street – for a fee – will write out 'scripts' (prescriptions), which have a very good street value. The prescribed drugs can be used as effectively as the original, and often some surplus can be exchanged or sold for more. Alcoholics can always find a drying-out clinic where their every need is filled – a psychiatrist to discuss their woes at length, nurses to cater for every whim and visiting friends or bribable staff to ensure a constant supply of booze.

We have not discussed the symptoms of addiction, except for

lying, self-deception and loss of moral values. A clear symptom is immaturity and irresponsibility. These addictions appear to arrest emotional development, even to reverse it. Addicts, creating havoc and confusion in their wake, behave like spoiled five year olds. They want what they want when they want it. They are also skilled manipulators – able to turn every situation to their advantage – the advantage, needless to say, being another drink, drug or bet. Addicts are constantly short of money, time and temper. They are long on excuses, alibis and lies. They lose interest in ordinary things, in other people and the 'real' world. Above all, they lose their own self-respect.

It should be remarked that addicts – particularly of drugs and alcohol – are often very clever at persuading not only their medical advisors, but also their families, that they are really suffering from either great problems in living or have other disorders such as severe depression, manic depression, paranoia, or a host of other ailments. This may even be true. But until they stop using the drug or drink, there is little likelihood of effective treatment. It is medically established that alcoholism mimics all manner of other ' illnesses in its symptoms. It also creates them. Many alcoholics and addicts suffer from claustrophobia, agoraphobia and acute depressive symptoms – all of which miraculously disappear, over time, when they cease to use the drug. But not until then.

As to the 'problems in living' – forget it. If like many other distraught parents, you allow them to con you into sending them away (Kibbutzes are quite popular), it's unlikely to make any difference. The problem lies in themselves, not in where they live. There are drugs, alcohol or gambling everywhere, and the addict who hopes to find geographical escape is kidding himself, and you too.

Inside addicts a constant battle rages. They are full of fear, anger and self-pity. They are often swamped with guilt, remorse and terror of impending insanity or suicide. These feelings come out sometimes in anger, sometimes in depression. But when the craving strikes, the addict is at its mercy.

And so, dear parent, are you, unless you are aware of what

you are up against, and willing to take out the kind of personal insurance policy which this book is all about.

What Can You Do About It?

In theory there is not too much you can do about it, because all the evidence points to the fact that the addict will not stop practising his or her adiction until they have had enough, until they are 'sick of being sick'. The addict has to want to stop. The addict also needs help to stop.

In theory you can do nothing. In practice, you can close all the doors except the ones to recovery and health. You can arm yourself with facts, addresses of treatment centres, information about recovery programmes – and make sure these are known to your dearly loved addict – but ultimately the decision for life or for death is theirs.

I am now going to add another paradox to the already confused picture. Addiction is certainly an illness. But it is an illness unlike any other. If your child had cancer or heart disease, diabetes or appendicitis, you would very properly run round helping and fetching and carrying, foreseeing and fulfilling every wish. The treatment for addiction is the *exact reverse*.

In the matter of addiction, it can be stated with absolute and categorical truth that KINDNESS CAN KILL.

The parent who gives a child money or goods which can be exchanged for the object of addiction is in fact giving them death.

The longer a parent knowingly protects an addict, the more destruction that addict can wreak upon him or herself.

Recovered addicts admit with total honesty that they were always supported or protected by someone, usually a parent, sometimes a grandparent, sister, brother, lover or other relative. As long as the support lasted, they continued with their habit – whatever that habit was. Recovered addicts acknowledge that while using, they did not have 'loved ones', they had 'hostages'.

Support or protection comes in many guises. It can come in terms of direct gifts, 'loans', or free board and lodging. It can come in helping them pay off bad debts, fines, or getting them

16

out of unpleasant situations. It can come in lying and covering up for them. All this is known as 'enabling'. It might also, with justice, be called 'disabling'.

Over and over again recovered addicts can be heard to say that they only took the decision to do something about their addiction when the protection was withdrawn, when they were forced to confront the full reality of what their lives had become.

This is what parent-power is all about. When parents are no longer willing to be 'hostages', no longer mirror the addiction, are no longer subjects or objects of bribery, blackmail or threats, then the addict begins to feel the ground slide away beneath his or her feet. In this way your addict can be allowed to reach the moment of truth known in many circles as the 'rock bottom'. This is the moment when the addict makes a personal decision to do something positive about his or her addiction.

But how to do it? How to retrieve this parent-power? First of all you need knowledge. You need to become aware not only of the symptoms but also of the tell-tale signs that kids may often leave lying about, whether because they are too out of order to clear up, or whether they are deep down hoping you'll find out. You've also got to be armed with information about drugs and the results of using them. It's high time we opened up the whole freemasonry of the drug scene and let in some air. Part of the risk-kick is leaving around evidence and dropping phrases that idiot parents don't understand or notice. O.K. When this book gets into their hands there'll doubtless be a few new ones. But many parents – even those with children knee-deep in drugs – do not recognise signs as evident (to a user) as the combination of a mirror and razorblade.

So now we are going to get some knowledge – and after that, action. As you read on you will learn techniques for breaking out of the 'hostage' situation, for recovering your self-confidence and self-respect. You will discover that there are ways in which you can get help and support to win back control of your own life – and in doing so, help your child towards asking for the help they need. What is suggested may cause you to do quite a lot of re-thinking about what you are doing and how you are acting. But this way lies hope – perhaps the only hope there is.

But equally, parents who recover from their child's addiction, grow in grace and in health. Just as the illness of addiction is contagious, and infects the whole family, so too does returning health. Recovery is catching.

If you want to see recovering addicts/alcoholics in the mass, take yourself off to where they foregather. You will certainly be within reach of a meeting of Alcoholics Anonymous or Gamblers Anonymous and with luck there might be a meeting of Narcotics Anonymous in your area. Unless you have a problem yourself, you may only go to an Open or a Public Meeting, but what you see and hear will certainly restore your faith in the possibilities of recovery for your son or daughter. You may not be ready to take that step yet. But bear it in mind. For it is important to realise that it is one thing to come off the drug but it is another to stay off it. The disease or illness of addiction is 'a chronic disorder with a tendency to relapse', as the American Medical Association Manual states. These organisations provide both instant treatment and continuous world-wide aftercare.

And if you want to see recovering families getting well, then find a meeting of Alanon (alcohol is the addiction) of Gamanon (for families of compulsive gamblers) or Families Anonymous (for drugs and related behaviour) if there is one in your area. There you will find hope and concrete help from the shared experiences of those who have been where you are.

But if you are not yet ready to admit your concern outside the pages of this book, just do what feels comfortable for yourself – and read on.

TWO

GETTING TO KNOW THE SCORE

A Table of Addiction

	Physical addiction	Psycho–logical addiction	Causes physical damage	Causes mental damage	Likely to lead to prison	Suicide risk
Alcohol	YES	YES	YES	YES	YES	YES
Marijuana	NO	YES	YES	YES	YES	NO
LSD	NO	NO	NO	YES	YES	YES
Heroin	YES	YES	YES	YES	YES	YES
Cocaine	YES	YES	YES	YES	YES	YES
Speed	YES	YES	YES	YES	YES	YES
Valium	YES	YES	YES	YES	NO	YES
Gambling	NO	YES	NO	NO	YES	YES
Work	NO	YES	NO	NO	NO	YES
Nicotine	YES	YES	YES	NO	NO	NO
Food (anorexia)	YES	YES	YES	YES	NO	YES
Solvents	YES	YES	YES	YES	YES	YES

Alcohol smells. Anorexia is easily detectable. Gambling is something most people know about. But many parents are unfamiliar with drugs, even those which are fairly commonly used by young people, so here follows a list of the most available drugs and an outline of their likely effects, both short and long term. Also how they are used. It is important to remember that all the drugs affect individuals differently. I have known people for whom cannabis is no more remarkable than nicotine, but a young recovered addict told me the effect of cannabis on him was catastrophic. He often became prey to appalling paranoid fear.

But it is important to have information. So in order to take some of the mystery out of the drug scene, you can now get acquainted with some of the vocabulary. You may know some already. The list is not – and never could be – complete. New terms are coined all the time in different groups all round the world. As soon as this book appears, some will be dropped like hot cakes and new ones invented. But some are pretty standard. You may as well know them.

Some Common Terms In The Drug Scene In The Eighties

Acid	LSD
Barbs	Barbiturates
Billy	Speed (abbreviation for 'Billy Whizz')
Blow	Cannabis
Bush	Cannabis
Bust (N or V)	Interference by police

Chasing the dragon Inhaling heroin
Chillum (or chillom) Pipe for smoking cannabis

Chinese	Heroin
Clean	Off drugs
Clucking	Coming off heroin, having withdrawals
Coke	Cocaine
Comedown	Effect of coming off speed or similar

Dragon	Heroin (see chasing)
Dope	Cannabis mainly, but sometimes heroin
Downer	Any drug that dispels anxiety or depresses e.g. alcohol, valium, barbiturates
Drop	To ingest or the ingestion of a drug

Fix	To inject or an injection of a drug or combination
Flashback	Momentary return to bad trip from hallucinogen

Free-basing	See under 'Cocaine'
French Blues	Amphetamine Sulphate
Gauze	Metal piece used in chillum or pipe
Gear	Drugs
Grass	Cannabis
Gouching out	After too much heroin, user becomes sleepy, eyes close, head drops & occasional effort is made to appear conscious
H	Heroin
Hash	Cannabis resin
Head	Anyone who takes drugs
Henry	Heroin
Herb (pronounced 'erb')	Rasta for cannabis
High	Out of your mind on a drug, euphoric
Hit	The sensation created by use of drug, e.g. injection of heroin
Horse	Heroin
Jack up	Inject substance
Joint	Cigarette laced with cannabis
Junk	Heroin
Junkie	A heroin addict
Kick	Stop using drug of choice
Magic Mushrooms	Psylocybins, powerful hallucinogen growing wild in fields, woods etc.
Mainlining	Injecting
O.D.	Lethal overdose of drug – i.e. death or near miss
Peaking	A high point in drug experience
Pinned-out	Dilated pupils
Popping	Injecting into skin or muscle (not vein)
Pot	Cannabis
Pothead	A person stoned on cannabis most of the time

Resin	Product of marijuana
Roach	Cardboard filter for drugged cigarette
Rush	A wave of drug-induced euphoria
Safi	Cotton or muslin scarf for chillum
Score (v)	To get a drug
Shooting up	Injecting into vein
Skag	Heroin
Skin	A cigarette paper
Smak	Heroin
Snort	To sniff through the nose
Snowball	Mixture of heroin and cocaine
Spaced out	Intoxicated on drugs
Speed	Amphetamine
Speedball	Mixture of heroin and speed
Spikes	Hypodermic needles
Splif	A cannabis cigarette
Stoned	Intoxicated through use of drugs
Stash	Drugs
Straight	A person who does not use, or has stopped using drugs
Tea	Old fashioned term for cannabis
Toke	To draw on a joint (verb) or the joint (noun)
Toot	To snort or sniff cocaine
Turkey 'cold turkey'	Coming off drugs without use of other drugs. Skin often goes goose-pimply and sensitive, hence the term
Upper	Any drug that makes you 'high' e.g. amphetamines, cocaine
Weed	Cannabis
Whizz	Speed
Wrap	Envelope of heroin (see illustration) or heroin in cling film

Drugs – and the Denial Game

Part of the problem of addiction is that one of the presenting symptoms is lying. Denial is the name of the game. It isn't only the addict who denies. It is also the parent who wants to avoid facing the truth about a beloved child. But ignorance can only make things worse – and possibly jeopardise your child's life.

The effects of drugs are very varied, as you will discover from the following pages. It can be extremely hard for a parent to decide whether their child is actually using drugs, or whether odd behaviour may simply be a singularly nasty outbreak of adolescence. How can you tell?

The answer is you can't. There is no doubt, however, that children who are behaving in very troublesome ways are more likely to be at risk. Unhappy, disgruntled, bored children are vulnerable to the instant escape offered by drugs, especially since they are now so readily to hand in the youth culture. They may also be troublesome and troubled because they are using drugs.

You may already have talked about drugs to your child. Chances are they have either denied all use or admitted to 'having tried it once or twice' or, 'just having a joint now and then', at parties and so on.

This is where our own parents really had it made. There were only 'drugs' – spoken of in hushed whispers – and nobody ever clapped eyes on a junkie.

The marijuana culture has changed all that. Though not legal, for twenty years it has been publicised, glamorised and trivialised. If you're over forty and you've tried cannabis, you are quite rare. Most parents don't even know what it looks like, or what its effects can be.

But because of its glamorous and quasi-respectable associations, marijuana is a convenient catch-all if admission of drug use cannot be avoided. Almost any user of any drug will admit, if pressed, to using cannabis now and then.

Because marijuana is both the baseline and the borderline for drug-taking, we'll look at it first and in some detail.

Cannabis

Majijuana is an Inebriating Narcotic

'Young people smoking marijuana together are peaceful, loving and sensitive to others' feelings. People don't put each other down. No competition. Much greater eye contact. Music is appreciated more since most of the good rock bands have been influenced themselves by this drug. In heightened states of awareness telepathy is possible and there's a sense of unity with mankind all over the world and barriers like countries, states and other commercial propositions cease to be relevant. It's an enjoyable experience because the past and future are not now, are they? – and now is the happiest time of your life. That's what taking marijuana starts out to be.' (John C.)

Marijuana is a plant, which flourishes in a warm climate but can be grown in this country and often is. The plant produces (harmless) food, hemp for sails and rope and fabric as well as substances used in medicine and some religious ceremonies. The dried leaves produce the 'weed' or 'grass'. The buds and top leaves provide the resin which is most potent and is scraped, or pressed into cakes which vary in colour. They can be brown, black, pink, red or greenish yellow.

Cannabis is an hallucinogen. It is also a narcotic. It changes perception. However its usage has to be learnt. Few people take to it the first time they try it, any more than alcohol is naturally enjoyed by humans.

Also known as 'pot', 'dope', 'hash', 'ganga', 'hemp', 'bush' and by many other names, cannabis is not thought to be physically addictive. It can, however, be psychologically addictive. Stopping the use of cannabis will rarely, if ever, produce physical withdrawal symptoms – but it may involve a person in giving up either a way of life, or a group of friends and above all, a way of escape from anxiety and the here-and-now reality.

Physical and Behavioural Symptoms of Cannabis Use

1. Smell on person and clothing – a distinctive, heavy 'grass' smell.
2. Flushed cheeks and bloodshot eyes soon after use. If challenged, this will probably be explained away by 'coughing fit', 'slight cold developing', 'smoke in eyes' etc.
3. Use of joss sticks (for covering up smell).
4. Lack of enthusiasm actually to DO anything. Big talk, little action.
5. Cannabis users are generally quiet, gentle and non-violent. Tend to despise alcohol and heroin. Hate to be called 'junkies' (until and unless they decide to experiment themselves).
6. Take pessimistic view of 'straight' world and strongly dislike the police. Much given to denying the value-systems and integrity of all institutions and any person who doesn't use, particularly if that person is over twenty five.
7. Increased appetite, especially for 'midnight munchies' – cereals, toast and lots of sugar and sweets.
8. Remarkable interest in the geography and lifestyles of countries such as India, Morocco and Jamaica – all places where cannabis is widely used and as much a part of the scenery as drinking is in Britain.

For rolling a 'joint', 'splif', 'number' (old fashioned 'reefer'), the following things are required: cigarette paper, tobacco, some marijuana in any form and a good rolling board or smooth surface. Most commonly used are shiny record sleeves.

Stick three cigarette papers ('skins') together to make it longer for passing round the room. Put tobacco down the centre of the papers and sprinkle or crumble marijuana evenly along the tobacco and roll papers around it into tube shape. Insert a small, lightly-rolled cardboard strip (a 'roach') into the mouth-end (to stop the tobacco and marijuana being sucked into mouth). The 'joint' is now ready to be ignited and passed around, if in company. Intoxication – called 'being stoned' – follows.

Tell-tale signs of Cannabis Use

1. Cigarette papers with the cardboard top torn off.
2. Cigarette packets with pieces torn off (for roaches).
3. Unsmoked cigarettes ripped open for tobacco.
4. In ash trays, very long roll-up dog-ends with cardboard filters.
5. Small pieces of loose tobacco on books, or record covers.
6. Loose grass seeds.
7. Small pieces of cling film.
8. Ripped up bits of cardboard.
9. Small plastic see-through bank bags (about 3 inches square) or similar (for containing cannabis).

How a chillum (chillom) is used:

A chillum is for smoking marijuana.

Tobacco plus hash or grass (resin or leaf) are mixed in a bowl, occasionally with a drop of water. The cigarettes are often toasted before the tobacco is used. The chillum is wrapped in a muslin or cotton scarf knows as a 'safi'.

After a ceremonial lighting, the chillum is held in both hands and smoked.

Tell-tale signs of chillum use are:

1. Roasted cigarette papers.
2. Interesting chillums (see illustration).
3. Round fine mesh metal 'gauzes', about the size of a five pence piece, blackened.
4. Small cone-shaped stones with bevelled edges about ¾ inch high (2 cm).
5. Cotton or muslin scarves stained with tobacco.
6. Small mixing bowls with bits of tobacco in.

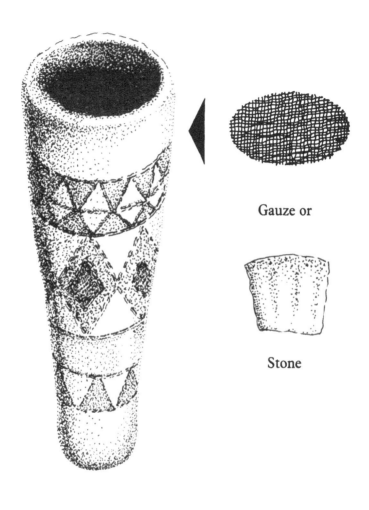

Gauze or

Stone

Chillum or Chillom

Plain or ornate, made from wood, clay or ceramic.
Actual size.

Notes:
Cannabis is also eaten in cakes – occasionally. ('Too much hassle, man').

Cannabis can be filtered through water-pipes. If these are around, and have water in, they are in use!

Unless a person is into dope, there is little point in collecting unusual small pipes – or large complicated water pipes.

Don't Be Bamboozled

Non addictive?

Cannabis users frequently insist that the drug is safer and better than alcohol (which is legal), and that it is not physically addictive. However alcohol is addictive only to certain people. Alcoholism occurs in *people* not in bottles. Many people can drink moderately without becoming alcoholics. Cannabis is known to induce psychological addiction in some people.

No physical effects?

Cannabis users claim it is not physically damaging. Recent research shows that the use of marijuana causes brain damage (short and long term), resulting in loss of memory, slow-down of learning process and dulling of perception. It causes progressive brain atrophy leading to shrinkage of the cerebral structures, including loss of fluid in the inner brain cavity – this fluid being replaced by air.

Even moderate use of marijuana (about three cigarettes a week) interferes with production of RNA and DNA in body cells of up to 41 per cent of new cell production. Marijuana also interferes with the body's immune response system and users suffer significant chromosome breaks.

Cannabis affects both male and female reproductive systems. In a recent test, sperm counts of 35 per cent of male cannabis users were found to be so low as to render them sterile.

Marijuana causes more damage to lungs than tobacco. (For fuller information on this, see reading list.)

A good, natural drug?

Given half an ear, the cannabis user will recount at length and in detail the spiritual and sensory delights induced by the drug. The user is unlikely to dwell on its less pleasant aspects. These include loss of will-power, motivation, concentration, affection for the non-user (including family), learning ability and span of attention. Quite a few losses, you will observe. It can, and does, cause apathy, personality deterioration and anti-social behaviour. Paranoia (irrational fear) is a not uncommon consequence of the use of this drug.

Doesn't lead to other drugs?

Defenders of cannabis (i.e. your misbehaving youngsters) will protest strongly that its use does not lead to the use of other drugs. Every former user of marijuana answered this question with the unanimous, if inelegant response, 'bullshit'.

The fact is that an adult, with an intact personality, a stable lifestyle and an established career, may find an occasional illicit 'joint' at a party non-addictive. It will be unlikely to lead to exploration of other drugs.

But children, adolescents and people with underlying personality disorders are very vulnerable. The use of marijuana does not *have* to lead to the use of other drugs, but it frequently does, notably in young people. In Germany it is known as 'the drug of introduction'.

In 1976 a survey was taken of marijuana users, with a control group of non-users. Of those who smoked marijuana three times a week, 52 per cent used amphetamines (speed), 51 per cent used LSD, 44 per cent used cocaine, 24 per cent used opiates, 20 per cent used barbiturates and 28 per cent used tranquillizers. None of these substances were used by the non-marijuana users.

Almost any heroin addict will inform you that the first drug used was cannabis. That this is generally true is borne out by a US study of 367 heroin addicts, all but four of whom had used marijuana before using heroin.

There are several reasons for this. The first is the hoary old one about being in touch with people on the wrong side of the law. This is only partly true. Introduction to marijuana is usually effected by an offer from a friend to 'share a joint' – to share, in fact, an experience which the friend has found enjoyable.

However, regular use certainly does put the child or adolescent in touch with more disturbed and damaged people, as well as a whole new sub-culture. If they want more cannabis they may have to 'score' for themselves. If they cannot get it through a friend, they may have to approach a dealer. The dealer will at some time offer other drugs.

Thus, the following things can occur:

1. Excitement at the prospect of a new experiment with 'one's head and heart', as a user put it.
2. Encouragement from friends.
3. Lowered judgement and will-power. After using cannabis it may be difficult to refuse to go along with the rest.
4. Enjoyment of varied effects given by alternating and changing drugs. Known combinations are 'speedball' (heroin & speed) or 'pills and Pils' (amphetamines & alcohol).

'When I started using marijuana other people's feelings were very apparent and interesting to me – but ultimately I only was aware of my *own* problems and feeling'. (John C., after six years of usage. Aged twenty).

Hallucinogens

LSD (d-lysergic acid diethylamide) – Acid

This is the most potent mind-altering substance known. On LSD people have what are known as 'trips'.

A vast amount has been written about the psychological and neurological effects of acid, but its precise effects on the human system are still not entirely clear. It is a chemical, not an organic drug.

Certainly many people have had 'trips' which they declare to be irreplaceably valuable. Sense impressions are heightened, time appears to stand still, everything seen, heard or felt appears to happen as for the first time. They report a sense of total awe and wonder. In some ways an acid trip can be likened to a short cut to the mystic's state of grace.

But short cuts usually have to be paid for.

Bad trips are indeed bad. The 'goodness' or 'badness' of a trip is unquestionably related to the person's personality, problems and the company he or she is in when LSD is taken.

People with personality problems are in grave risk when they use LSD. There is a clear correlation between many of the effects of LSD and the states induced by schizophrenia, sensory deprivation, and *delirium tremens*. LSD does not create dependence. Toleration builds up (i.e. a user needs more and more to get a 'trip') – but in a fairly short time, interest in the drug diminishes. However unstable people have used acid too often with extremely serious results, not excluding permanent mental impairment ('acid heads'). (For fuller information on this see reading list).

How LSD is taken

Acid usually comes in two forms. Either in very small pills, known as 'tabs', or even smaller pills, 'mikes' (because LSD dosage is in micromilligrams). The smaller pills are about the size of a saccharine tablet.

The second method is by swallowing a small square (about 1 cm.) of blotting paper cut from an A4 sheet, which has been carefully marked out so that each dosage is exact. The blotting paper is impregnated with acid, and may or may not contain either overall designs to the buyer's choice, or each square may have a special design on it.

Tell-tale signs of LSD use

There are almost none. Someone on a 'trip' is going to try and avoid parents as much as possible, and although the user will feel strange, the parent will probably observe nothing very odd about the user's appearance.

You might notice very dilated (expanded) pupils and extreme sensitivity – but getting someone to go and stand near a light or a window while you look into their eyes is really not on. You are very unlikely to find sheets of blotting paper lying about or small pills.

'Most of my trips were refreshing and enjoyable experiences', reports a former user, 'but finally I had two bad trips. Even with these I learnt something – and that was not to take any more, because LSD is a chemical and the drug is in my own mind, and so is the experience.' Excessive use of LSD can cause permanent psychiatric disorder.

Other addicts, especially those who have used LSD in parallel with other drugs, suffer in other ways. The phenomenon known as the 'flashback' can occur for many months or even years after a bad trip. This is a sudden return to the experience of the bad trip, and causes great fear and anguish.

Magic Mushrooms (Psylocybins)

Also known as 'liberty caps', these mushrooms flourish from late summer to the first frost, in fields and woods in various parts of the country. In south Wales, a Psylocybin Festival is held in early autumn to which youngsters (and ageing hippies) repair in search of the 'trips' afforded by this hallucogenic plant. (This festival follows 'Stoned Henge').

Method of use: Magic mushrooms can be ingested in many forms. Just as they are, or immersed in hot water like tea, or cooked in anything (on omelette?). The dosage can be effective with as few as one, as many as 200. However the mushrooms contain other substances and cause stomach pains if taken in quantity.

Tell-tale signs

You might find a bag of the mushrooms – but it's not likely.

One mother was appalled when her son came home with his

pockets full of the mushrooms wanting her to 'share' the marvellous experience with him. He was visibly inebriated, disorientated and unable to walk straight. It was evident that he had ingested many mushrooms. This mother's experience is probably uncommon. Like most drug taking, mushroom eating is normally kept away from 'straight' society. However the fact that the fungi grew in a nearby park, free for any to find, probably made the deluded boy imagine they were more 'acceptable' to a parent.

Parents coping with youngsters on drugs often listen and try to understand what their youngsters are on about. One recurrent phrase is that such and such a drug is 'organic' – meaning, in their terms, natural and healthy.

It's not much of an answer, and it won't probably get through to your kid, but it might make you a bit easier to retort tartly that deadly nightshade, foxglove and the sweet smelling lily of the valley are also 'organic' plants. The fact that something grows out of the earth does not, in fact, make it healthy for human consumption.

The effects of magic mushrooms are similar to those of LSD – and so are the long term consequences.

Powders and Pills

Speed (Amphetamine Sulphate)

Until quite recently, speed was acceptable to the vast majority of young drug takers only in tablet form. There was a wariness about the use of powders, because of their associations with the so-called 'hard drugs' – heroin and cocaine.

In pill form aphetamine sulphate was normally coloured blue – hence the names 'blues' and 'French blues'. However other types of speed were also common and are still available today. These are 'dexies' (small yellow pills), 'black bombers', 'black and whites', 'green and browns' (these are all capsules in the named colours).

Amphetamine powder is crystalline, rather like castor sugar

with which it is often mixed. It is sold by the gramme or part thereof. A gramme will provide fifteen 'lines' and would fill about three quarters of a teaspoon.

How Amphetamine Sulphate is Used

The powder is usually purchased in small envelopes folded like this:

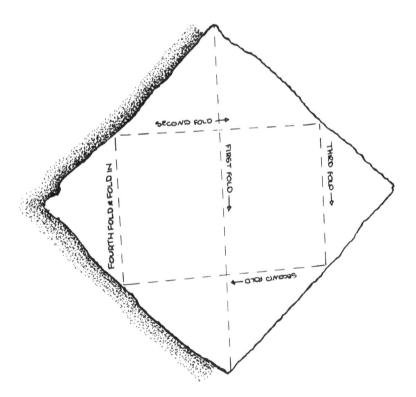

Powders
Heroin, Cocaine, Sulphate 'speed'.
Actual size.

1. Snorted: a small amount of the powder is crushed and chopped with a blade on a mirror or glass surface to eliminate the crystals. It is then divided (again with the blade) into a line – or as many lines as partakers. A finely rolled bank note or drinking straw is then used to sniff the powder into the user's nose.
2. Drunk: the powder can be dissolved in water and drunk. The effect is slightly slower than for snorting.
3. Injected: dissolved in water, speed can be injected. This has immediate effect. For description of method, see sections on barbiturates and heroin.

Tell-tale Signs

1. A mirror or hard shiny surface, such as glass.
2. A razor blade or very finely honed knife.
3. A tightly rolled bank note or drinking straw.
4. Small piece of paper (about 7cms, or 2½ inches square), with folds as illustrated.
5. Hypodermic syringe and needles.

Physical and Behavioural Symptoms of Speed Use

1. Hyperactivity, inability to sleep, wandering round house all night.
2. Fidgety, jumpy, nervous, excitable movements.
3. Sometimes dilation of the pupils of the eyes.
4. Rapid, rambling, repetitive speech.
5. Sudden enthusiasms – which die equally suddenly.
6. Very heavy cigarette smoking and/or chewing of gum.
7. Need for a great deal of liquid – tea, coffee, anything.
8. Frequent sniffing – without symptoms of the common cold.
9. Diminished or non-existent appetite.
10. Inability to concentrate for more than a few moments at a time.

After prolonged or heavy use:

11. Occasional dizziness.
12. Blotchy skin, drained pallid appearance.
13. Swollen lips with a blackish deposit at corners of mouth and sometimes on the lips themselves.
14. Rapid decay of teeth.

'Speed kills'. That is the verdict of all the former users and recovered addicts with whom I have talked.

It is also agreed that speed is the most subtle as well as the most dangerous of drugs, not least because its pharmaceutical application and legal classification make it appear mild – even safe, to the gullible youngster. Yet its effects are both long-term and horrific. It generates instant enthusiasm and energy – but it bankrupts the body, mind and spirit. It uses up all reserves. 'Amphetamines stretch you to the point that you snap,' said a former heavy drug user. He continued, 'It's the nastiest drug on earth, because initially it's one of the nicest. But the effects are devastating, draining. You don't notice how affected you've been by it for a long time afterwards. At least a year after heavy use before you really notice how sick you've been.'

The cyclist Simpson who died from a heart attack in the Olympics, from using amphetamine sulphate, is only one of the most publicised casualties of this drug. Many youngsters have also incurred heart attacks and even death from using speed. Some heavy users, withdrawn without medical care, do not survive the shock of amphetamine psychosis, described earlier, and have to remain permanently institutionalised.

Sleepers and Downers (Barbiturates and Tranquillizers)

Now we open a real can of worms. Barbiturates were described in The Lancet as long ago as 1954 as 'a true drug of addiction' but were still available on ordinary (and even 'repeat') prescriptions until very recently. However the medical profession has now taken steps to put its house in order and barbiturates are presently prescribed only in exceptional cases.

This does not stop the kids from getting hold of 'barbs'. Some are supposedly brought in from abroad, but anyone in the know can usually put the finger on a medical practitioner who is either (a) unscrupulous (b) old (c) or addicted and who will – for a consideration – write out a script/prescription.

However the place of barbiturates has been largely superceded by tranquillizers and sleeping pills which, as we all know, can be found in almost any home.

Like barbiturates, tranquillizers and sleeping pills are now being unmasked as the dangerous and addictive drugs they so often are.

However, just as it took the doctors years to come to terms with the dangers of barbiturates, it looks like taking a long time for the doctors to take proper action about 'tranx'.

But let us not start casting blame, neither on the medical profession, who only try to help (however misguidedly sometimes), nor on the pharmaceutical firms, who not only want to make money, but would prefer to make it ethically, nor on ourselves for demanding and using them.

The problem is really both deeper and simpler.

It is that, as a society, we have all got into the habit of thinking that tension, pain and sleeplessness are in themselves both bad and unnecessary. Which, if you look at it another way, is quite insane.

If I've got no job, no prospects and a family of kids to feed, sure I've got reasons for being tense and uptight and in pain. *If I choose to*. I can go to the surgery and get a hundred valium or librium or something and knock myself silly – but the problem will remain with me. Unless I've got my marbles there is no way I'm going to be able to take the necessary steps to make life more bearable, am I?

If my parent or dearest friend dies in an accident, I need to grieve. The pain of grief can be a healing gift. If I do not come to terms with the sadness and anguish of death or disaster when it happens, these feelings will lie in wait in the deep cupboards of my heart, and at the next crisis will leap out and overwhelm me.

And sleeplessness? Well, did *you* ever hear of anybody dying from lack of sleep? The body takes the sleep it needs. Accept a few 'White Nights'. Read a good book or watch a video. You won't fall apart. Your body will adjust – you probably think you need more sleep than you do. Remember Churchill? He only needed 4 hours a night.

But you almost certainly *have* heard of plenty of people who died from overdoses of tranquillizers or sleeping pills, usually taken together with alcohol.

The other way of looking at pain – and sleeplessness – is that it is there for a purpose. It is there to show us that we need to do something about our lives. I know it sounds hard, but pain can be used as an opportunity for growth. I do not intend to go into this here and now, but it needs thinking about, because tranquillizers and sleeping pills can be found in almost every home.

Kids use them. 'Moggies' and 'mandies', valium and librium are all useful when nothing else is around. They're good mixers too. Too much speed? Add a little valium – and you won't go right over the top.

The difficulty of coming off many tranquillizers and sleeping pills has been discussed (see page 11). The effect of barbiturates and tranquillizers is primarily to relieve anxiety. They are known as 'the escapers' drugs'.

Method of Use of Barbiturates (notably Blue Bombs) and Tranquillizers

1. Capsules: swallowed.
2. Injection: capsules can be opened and the powder mixed with water (which should be sterile but rarely is) and injected in either vein or muscle, as for heroin. This method frequently caused death because the powder may not be properly dissolved and abscesses can form which poison the whole system.

Cocaine

Cocaine is a powerful stimulant, which oddly enough also contains potent anaesthetic properties. Because of the latter, the flesh it touches is likely to suffer local damage. Hence the destruction of the bridge of the nose suffered by coke-snorters. Some users' nostrils are also destroyed, after excessive use. Its effect is primarily as an 'upper' – as is speed – the opposite effect to that of heroin and alcohol, both of which are basically 'downers'.

Cocaine comes from the leaves of the coca plant, originally grown in the Andes. It used to be the 'secret' ingredient in Coca Cola.

As with speed, cocaine produces instant energy, action, creativity – but at a high cost. Like speed, it enables the user to pillage his or her last resources, and, like speed, it is paid for in equal depths of depression and exhaustion.

Cocaine is, quite wrongly, believed to be non-addictive. It is extremely addictive, both physically and psychologically.

The high price of cocaine, even today, makes it the classiest form of self-destruction in terms of emotional and actual bankruptcy.

Physical and Behavioural Symptoms of the Use of Cocaine

It is not easy to detect behavioural changes in cocaine users – if they only use cocaine. Generally they appear to be somewhat manic-depressive – and not a few coke addicts have persuaded their families and medical practitioners that this is what their problem is. Addicts (of all kinds) are experts at fooling people. Only when they stop using, do they recognise that the only people they've really fooled are themselves. It is the addict who pays the piper ... and heavily, in more than one sense.

In youngsters, the pattern is similar to that for speed, but marginally less dramatic.

1. Great enthusiasm, nervous energy, cheerfulness – then
2. Depression, exhaustion and lack of energy.
3. Stealing.
4. Lying.
5. Frequent sniffing – with or without the common cold.
6. More stealing.
7. (After protracted use) damage to nose as described.
8. Yet more stealing.

Cocaine users, unlike heroin addicts, often prefer company to solitude. Cocaine appears to make people gregarious as well as open-handed and generous. They cheerfully offer a 'line' or a smoke to anyone who is around – which explains in part the frequent financial bankruptcies of cocaine addicts.

Method of Using Cocaine

1. It can be 'snorted' – as described for speed.
2. It can be inhaled in cigarettes to heighten the effects of snorting, but this is rare among teenagers. It does not require all the trappings necessary for cannabis smoking.
3. It can be smoked – for which purpose a chemical process known as 'freebasing' must take place. This means dissolving the impure cocaine (it is almost always impure when bought) in a test tube of ammonia or soda bicarbonate. The cocaine will sink to the bottom. This residue, now 100% pure cocaine, can be smashed up and smoked in a hubbly bubbly (water pipe).
4. It can be injected, mixed with water (see under heroin).

Tell-tale signs

1. As for speed – mirror or glass and razor blade or sharp knife.
2. The utensils as described above for freebasing. It is unlikely that many teenagers living at home will be found to use this method of taking cocaine.
3. Hypodermic syringes and needles.
4. Envelope, as illustrated.

Heroin

This is the most widely feared of all drugs and there are many who believe that the only outcome of heroin use is death.

This is not the case. Heroin users, like users of any other drug, can recover. Alcohol kills, speed kills – almost all the drugs mentioned here can kill – but from any drug or combination, recovery is possible and does in fact happen. The long term physical effects of heroin use are actually less damaging than those created by abuse of alcohol, if the user lives.

The damage caused to heroin addicts is for the most part done by the way of life. Serum hepatitis, skin infections, scarring and abscesses (from injections) – and of course, the ever-present possibility of overdosing are relatively common in the heroin sub-culture, as well as venereal disease, serious malnutrition and some liver damage. There is a great deal of literature on the chemical, neurological, physical and psychological effects and attributes of heroin, and I shall not attempt to expand here on these in any detail (see reading list).

Heroin is a derivative of opium. It is a narcotic. Very often the first use causes sickness, vomiting and nausea. But – as with all drugs – it is not always so. The first 'hit' can occasionally produce the unrivalled 'high', the unparalleled joy and release from anxiety that hooks the potential addict instantly. In general, it takes some determination to get addicted. Usually consistent use for two to three weeks is adequate.

But the mind and body are never fooled. So high the peaks, so low the depths. The heroin addict suffers without the drug in direct proportion to the pleasure taken by its use. It is even possible that the lows are as essential to the use as the highs – in some way the suffering assuages inner guilt – and makes possible the 'reward' of yet another high. Guilt however is always lying there in wait.

And the returns are diminishing. More heroin is needed to capture the first fine careless rapture. And in time the drug takes over so that all other concerns, all interests, all activity, all life is centred around getting and fixing, organising and using. Addiction is hard, unremitting work. It also involves enormous outlay, not just of money and time, but of initiative and cunning, to get the stuff, pay for it, avoid detection, evade the law – and in general to keep up an apparently ordinary front.

Heroin is known by many names. 'H', 'Henry', 'Horse', indeed by any noun beginning with an 'H' so that parents or other non-users will not understand references to the drug in conversation or over the telephone. However the most common name among users is 'smak'.

The interchangeability of drugs for addicts is particularly apparent in heroin users. Deprived of heroin, they will make do with pethidine, speed, diconal, morphine, DF 118, methadone, codeine linctus, alcohol or anything else.

How Heroin is Used

Heroin comes in two colours – white and brown.

White heroin is:

1. Snorted (as for cocaine)

Brown heroin is:

2. Inhaled. This is called 'chasing the dragon'. The brown powder is put on a piece of tin foil (creased) and the substance heated from underneath. This turns the powder into a brown drop of liquid which gives off vaporised fumes. Through a funnel the fumes are inhaled.
3. Both kinds of heroin can be injected. The brown powder is put in a teaspoon to which a couple of drops of citric acid or pure lemon juice (or more rarely, vinegar) are added. White heroin needs no citric acid. This is brought to the boil by heating the spoon underneath until the powder has dissolved. A little (sterile ??) water is usually added. Through a small filter (often a slice of cigarette filter) the liquid is drawn into a hypodermic. A check is made for air bubbles by upturning the syringe and tapping it.

A belt, scarf or tie is then used to make a tourniquet for the arm above whichever vein is planned to be used. This makes the veins stand up. (Until they collapse and another part of the anatomy is used). The vein is then injected ('hit') with the needle, and to ensure a vein has actually been hit, the plunger is slightly withdrawn. If blood shows, and mixes with the brownish liquid in the syringe, then the vein has been hit. If not, the process is repeated. When the user is certain to have found a vein, the heroin is slowly and fully released into the vein. The needle however remains in the vein and the plunger withdrawn to fill the syringe entirely with blood. This now gives what users call 'the rush'. Finally the plunger is pushed down and the new blood returned to the vein. This last process is called 'flushing'.

Overdoses (ODs) are common with injecting addicts, not only because of despair, but also because of mistakes. Someone who has been deprived of the drug may lose some of their tolerance and accidentally take more than the system can stand. A new supply or different dealer may provide heroin of a quality different from that which the user is accustomed to. The scenes of youngsters lying with blood on bathroom or bedroom walls and floors are not exaggerated.

When fully addicted, the heroin user will need to inject at 6 to 8 hourly intervals (at least), whereas a cocaine addict will need more of the stuff at intervals as short as half an hour to 40 minutes. For this reason, combinations are particularly damaging. 'With snowballs, my addiction needs were accelerated', said an addict, 'I had to deal as well as steal. My addiction was costing me £500 a week'. (That was at 1981 dealers' prices).

Track marks – red lines – can be seen inside elbows along the inside and outside of forearms, backs of hands – and particularly with girls, ankles. But by the time these appear, it is unlikely that a parent will be denying the problem any longer.

Physical and Behavioural Symptoms of Heroin Use

1. Change of behaviour. Aggression; cockiness.
2. Withdrawal from family life. 'I couldn't get through to her,' says a mother. 'She began isolating herself in her room.'
3. Diminishing appetite.

With increased heroin consumption, the symptoms increase too:

4. Lying.
5. Stealing.

6. Total isolation in room away from family.
7. Extreme thinness.
8. Beautiful, ethereal facial appearance and fragile look.
9. Rarely bothering with clothes. Perhaps two outfits. Seldom eccentric, since it is particularly important for heroin addicts to appear 'normal'.
10. No interest in family, social activities, or school.
11. Late night telephone calls.
12. Coming home late at night or not at all.
13. Staying in bed all day, watching T.V. if possible.
14. Refusing to lie in the sun or even, if possible, to go into sunlight (pinhead sized pupils – 'pinned-out' pupils – make bright light positively painful – hence the frequent use of dark glasses by addicts, and their preference for night and low lighting).
15. Always wearing long sleeves, high necklines and jeans (these cover injection marks).
16. Hate to be touched, hugged or embraced (highly sensitive skin – also the reason for simplified and few clothes).
17. Extreme aggression, irritability and insensitivity to others.
18. If addiction can be described as creating the Jekyll and Hyde syndrome (as it often is), then Hyde now predominates except when the addict wants something. Then Jekyll appears, all sweetness, promises and light – which lasts only until the demand has been met.
19. 'Gouching out' – sleepy appearance occasionally snapping awake.
20. Sweaty face (when withdrawing) and shaky hands.

Tell-tale signs

1. Untidy room.
2. Food plates and cups taken to room (heroin addicts need isolation). These accumulate under the bed.
3. Blackened teaspoons.
4. Lemons disappear from the kitchen. Sometimes found in addict's room. Or discarded packets of citric acid from chemist.

5. Glass or mirror (sometimes broken) and again, the razor blade with it.
6. Envelopes as for all powder drugs (as illustrated).
7. Small pieces of cling film.
8. Silver foil or takeaway foil tins bent as indicated and blackened on one side from flames.
9. Hypodermic syringes and needles.

Domestic Products

For reasons which sensible people will understand, I do not intend to expand very much on possible substances and their method of use in this section.

However there are certain well-known noxious substances, available in ordinary shops and accessible in most households, which misguided youngsters are known to tamper with – to their certain peril.

Codeine linctus is one such. Should you notice that your child is making free with this, it could indicate incipient addiction.

Solvents

Under this heading come ordinary lighter fuel (butane), dry cleaning fluids and various glues.

Solvents are said to be sniffed. In practice they are most commonly inhaled.

The immediate effect is generally a headrush, followed by tingling in the eyes, then at the back of the head followed by swift disorientation similar to extreme intoxication by alcohol.

'Soul destroying,' says a former user. 'You go quite out of your head. There's this contrast between ordinary life and the experience. That's what it's really about. Total disorientation. It numbs your mind so you can't even process your pain. Almost like kicking out at everything – sort of mindless head-butting against ... I don't know what? Yourself? The world? It's a sort of a short sharp wallop to the mind and body.'

One user, sitting one evening in front of the television while her parents were out, made free with almost a full canister of lighter fuel. 'The worst part was the end ... I felt my head was in a clamp and all my brains were being pushed in.' It's hard to believe but later, this girl was to use butane again. It was only one of many 'experiments' that she tried – and tried again, though by the time she was sixteen her drug of choice was alcohol. She continued to use alcohol (and anything else when it wasn't available) until she was 19. Today at 21 she has been drink and drug free for nearly 18 months, has a regular nine to five job, and lives in a small flat with another recovering user. Her mother and father had begun to use most of the practices suggested here.

The intoxicant effects of glue sniffing last slightly longer than the intoxication from butane. A mother describes how she found out about her son's use, 'He was using after school, and even at school sometimes. I thought he was drunk – but he didn't smell of it. Fortunately he got into trouble with the police – he was really scared and he's stopped since then. Today he's all right and getting back to normal.'

Behavioural Symptoms of Solvent Abuse

1. Red face (immediately after use).
2. Sitting with nodding head.
3. Slurred speech and drunken gait.
4. Vacant look in the eyes.
5. Aggressive, truculent behaviour (with hangover).
6. Possibility of violence, verbal if not physical (also with hangover).
7. Listlessness, apathy and lack of concentration.

Persistent use produces further symptoms:

8. Facial rash.
9. Running nose.

10. Poor muscle control.
11. At any stage, secretive behaviour and stealing are likely to happen.
12. Stomach pains and nausea are complained of.

Effects of Solvent Abuse

Solvent abuse kills. In 1983, official figures confirmed 59 deaths directly related to solvent abuse. That only accounts for the identified deaths. Solvent abuse leads to dangerous risk-taking and very aggressive behaviour, which may result in death but which are not recorded on death certificates – the only source of official statistics.

Consequences of solvent abuse include brain damage, heart attacks, kidney damage, fits, delusions and hallucinations. Death often happens through the user inhaling his own vomit.

Those sad youngsters who continue to inhale solvents can be easily recognised. They sit in frozen immobility, occasionally shaking their heads, perhaps, as one former user said to me, in the hope that the brain will work again. They speak, if at all, with difficulty. These are the sad cabbages who survive solvent abuse – if survival is the word.

Tell-tale Signs

1. Disappearance of any of the known substances.
2. Empty canisters, containers etc.
3. Plastic bag with glue remains.
4. Evidence of spilled glue sticking to furniture, floor or clothing.

Compulsive Gambling

The idea that compulsive gambling can be defined as a psychological addiction, hence an illness, may come as a shock to ordinary parents accustomed to a flutter on the Derby or a ticket in the local Scouts' raffle. But leaving aside 'heavy' and 'professional' gamblers, there are also people for whom gambling is as compulsive as heroin is for the addicted user. It is neither sinful nor weakness. It is an illness.

Gamblers Anonymous has helped many such people since 1957 (in the UK) but recently the tip has appeared of what is believed to be an iceberg of addicted youngsters. These are the fruit machine addicts. The kids who cannot stay away from the highs and lows they get in playing the machines.

Signs are quite difficult for parents to observe. Hugging the 'big secret' is one of the symptoms. In fact youngsters, with the cunning of all addicts, can often fool their parents for years. Dave got hooked on the machines at around 14. By 16 he knew every amusement arcade in his district. He managed to deceive his parents until he had to start stealing to feed his habit. When they found out, he still couldn't stop, nor could they stop him. At 18 he wrote to Gamblers Anonymous and by going regularly to meetings has been keeping away from the machines – and any other sort of gambling – for a year now.

Behavioural Patterns in Compulsive Gambling

1. Unaccounted for free time. Late homecoming from school or work.
2. Unaccounted for lack of money. Constant indebtedness.
3. Lack of friends. Usually sits alone in room at night.
4. Lack of interest in school or work or family affairs.
5. Hungry (lunch money spent on machines).
6. Lying.
7. Stealing, fraud, burglary.

Dave's habit was costing him £100 a week when he stopped. Two of the boys I talked to were awaiting serious court cases and they were both 19. The outcome for the compulsive gambler who does not get help to stop, will almost certainly be prison or suicide.

Alcohol – the legal drug of abuse

'I'd wake up in a cell, knowing nothing and ask 'what have I done this time?' said Judy (21). 'I can't deny it because I can't remember ... I've been on loads and loads of charges ... criminal damage, assault, threatening words and behaviour – don't know where they got that one about the words, – drunk and disorderly ... all over London I've paid fines.' Judy had already been in two women's prisons.

The idea that alcoholics are pathetic old men and women huddled under the arches, dies hard. In fact alcoholism or problem drinking, as some people prefer to call it, can start at any age and arrive either full-blown or grow slowly and insidiously. It can hit the schoolgirl of 14 or the chairman of the board at 60.

Alcoholics do not necessarily like the taste of liquor. They crave, however, what it does for them. What it does for them, eventually is lead to death, to prison or a psychiatric institution. The stages between are liable to be punctuated by breaking of family ties, losing friends, careers and jobs, prison charges, visits to psychiatrists and funny farms, throwing up every morning, the sweats, the shakes, the fears – 'Oh God, the fears' and finally total breakdown, physical, mental and emotional.

Some Behavioural and Physical Symptoms of Alcoholism

1. Obvious drunkenness, regularly or sporadically.
2. Fury if kept away from expected visit to pub.
3. Shortage of cash.
4. Lying about where cash goes.
5. Lying about amount drunk (either boasting of 'drinking everyone under the table', or the reverse, pretending to having drunk less than is true).
6. Defensiveness if challenged about drinking.
7. Denial of problem.
8. Aggressive or extremely withdrawn, secretive behaviour.

49

9. Dislike of getting physically too close to people (the smell tells).
10. Eating peppermints (in vain hope of disguising smell).
11. Hiding bottles (either full or empty).
12. 'Sneaking' drinks from the house – often replacing the liquid with water.
13. No friends (if a secret drinker).
14. All friends are drinkers (if a pub drinker).
15. Throwing up in the morning ('dry retching').
16. Shaky hands, when needing a drink particularly.
17. Trouble with the police.

It has been said that, 'if alcohol were invented today by a research chemist, it would be stringently controlled by law'. However it is an accepted, legal part of social (and often business) activity in this country and unquestionably a great many people can drink – even quite heavily – without becoming afflicted by the condition of alcoholism.

Families of problem drinkers suffer deeply. They, too, are damaged by the illness, they too learn tricks of manipulation and control, of lying, blackmail, covering-up and bribing. Above all they, like their sick child, all too often deny there is a problem at all.

It is very hard indeed to admit that your child is a drunk. But only by accepting the truth of that admission and acting on it, in the ways suggested here, is there any hope for early release for your child. Alcoholism is progressive. Things can only get worse until the alcoholic accepts the need for help in recovery. The 'rock bottom' was a term coined by alcoholics. It is possible to raise that 'rock bottom' so that your child can arrive at a decision to do something about his or her drinking without having to go through all the anguish and shame, degradation and despair that lies along the path to eventual self-destruction, the end product of alcoholism.

For that you are going to need all your parent-power.

Garbage Heads

In more than one treatment centre, those youngsters who use anything and everything are known as 'garbage heads'. Doctors say they are cross-addicted.

In fact, practically every sick addict is likely to be a garbage head if only because the drug of choice may not always be available. Some users/addicts start out with the understandable (if regrettable) intention of testing out the limits of their endurance, whether of pain or of mind. A highly articulate recovered addict, who had tried every substance he could discover, distinguished between what he called the mind-expanding substances and the mind-contracting substances. 'The sulphates, glue and gas are all mind-contractors,' he declared. 'A lot of kids think they're mind-expanders, like the hallucinogens, but they're not. They contract it. The escape drugs, the opiates and alcohol – they diminish pain, they don't really expand the mind.'

These are fine distinctions, and not everyone – user or scientist would necessarily agree with them. What is true is that once in the drug scene, it is rare for someone not to try other substances. A number even survive these perilous experiments and come through unscathed. Others cross what is known as the 'thin red line' – where the possibility of easily stopping merges into true addiction. Few addicts know, even in retrospect, when that line has been crossed. But all too often it is crossed for ever.

If addiction occurs, then any state of changed consciousness is better than facing the reality of the daily round. Whether the substances are called mood-altering, mind-altering or consciousness-changing, the fact that the user is 'somewhere else' is what is important. Even if that place is infinitely more painful, that is better than coping with school, work or just getting up in the morning.

For this reason, parents who are concerned that their kids may be experimenting with drugs would do well not to try to define too closely which drugs might be in question – in other words, the specific signs and symptoms I have outlined should be interpreted with discretion. Most successful recovery programmes accept as axiomatic that once an addict, always an addict. There can be no more 'social' drugging or drinking. Addiction is both progressive – and for ever.

For that reason, it can only ever be arrested, not cured. In many recovery progammes, notably those based on Alcoholics Anonymous, the addict or alcoholic is said to be, not recover*ed*, but recover*ing*. But recovery does happen – and that's what you need to hang on to. The hope of recovery and your own part in it. For parent-power is a major tool in getting your troubled child to ask for help.

THREE

THE NEED TO CHANGE

Clearly addiction creates havoc. It changes not only the user but also the family. Equally, some 'normal' adolescent rebellion can cause great unhappiness and turmoil, even when it is practised by a child who is not necessarily going to turn into a full-fledged addict. So something has got to change, unless the misery and despair is to engulf everyone. Because *you* have the potential for healing parent-power, it is *you* who will have to make the first changes – in yourself.

'Why should *I* change?' I hear you cry defensively. 'It's my child who is all the trouble ... bunking off school, getting stoned, bringing all those dreadful people into the house, having strange telephone calls in the middle of the night, staying in bed till all hours, refusing to get a job, demanding money, stealing from the house, getting into trouble with the law, telling barefaced lies, blackmailing me, always breaking promises ...' the list is endless. Take your pick.

What is clear is that your dear little baby, your delightful toddler, your lovable five-year old has changed out of all recognition.

But what about yourself? Are *you* the same cheerful, sunny person you used to be? Are *you* unchanged by all this? If you've been experiencing those emotions we just talked about, then for sure you are not the person you used to be when you were a new, proud parent and the world was your oyster.

Let's look at the ways parents express their unhappy emotions and see where we stand. Here is a very short list of what we shall call parental misbehaviour. Think about which ones apply to you.

Nagging ... Bullying ... Suspiciousness ... Complaining ...

Screaming ... Bribing ... Threatening ... Sarcasm ... Covering-up ... Lying ... Sneering ... Criticising ... Whining ...

Have you been aware of doing any of those things in the last twenty four hours? In the last week? Were you that sort of person ten years ago?

What I am getting at is that just as your child has changed, so have you. And not, it might seem for the better. Now unless you want to keep the situation as it is, or allow it to get worse, someone has to change. They're changing anyway .... but you have no power or control over how. But you *can* change yourself – you *have* got power over yourself. You can control your actions, your attitudes and your behaviour.

What is more, if you begin changing, there is no doubt that your misbehaving youngster is going to get a hell of a shock. The world will start looking a great deal different. Look at that list again. Can you say, with hand on heart, that any of that behaviour really got you anywhere? Has it in fact made your troublesome child less troublesome?

It has been said that 'insanity is doing the same things you've always done and expecting to get different results'.

No, I'm not saying you are insane, though you may well be half out of your mind with worry. In any case you are almost certainly more sane than your troubled teenager. For that reason, if no other, the change has to begin with you. It may indeed be the only hope left for your child's life.

Accepting Unacceptable Behaviour

The next positive step you can take is to stand back from the situation and start regarding your child as a person. By the time a child is thirteen (if not earlier) they know the difference between right and wrong. They know the kind of behaviour that is expected of them. Fifty years ago, they'd probably be leaving school, going out to work and helping to supplement the family budget. They can't do that now. They have to stay at school, under your roof, until they are sixteen or while they are still in education.

Nonetheless they *are* under your roof and protection. That means they have a responsibility to behave in the manner which you need for your own peace of mind and the tranquil running of your home. Is your child behaving in ways that you would not put up with from a visitor, another member of the family, or one of your friends?

It is not possible, as I said earlier, to be specific about what is OK and what is not. It is different in every family, for every parent. The point is, are *you* putting up with behaviour that is really unacceptable to you?

Only you know what you find unacceptable. Nobody outside can tell you. In one family it might be not coming in at an agreed time. In another it might be bashing the furniture around.

If you know in your gut that you *are* accepting unacceptable behaviour, start giving it some deep thought. Think about what you really expect to happen in your home. Sit down quietly and be realistic about it. It may be that you cannot bear people smoking cannabis in your home. You may wish to have the music turned off at midnight. You may decide you must have your son/daughter pay you X amount of money from their dole every week for food and board. You may think of any one of a hundred things – but when I say be realistic, I mean consider those matters over which you do have control. You cannot control what anybody does *outside* your home, but your home is yours – and inside it, you make the rules.

For a little while don't do anything about it, but bear in mind, and keep repeating like a mantra, the key to clearing a great deal of this mess: I DO NOT HAVE TO ACCEPT UNACCEPTABLE BEHAVIOUR.

Just keep saying it over to yourself and let it sink in. You will probably begin to recognise how far, over the weeks or months or years the behaviour in your home has deteriorated. You will understand just how your own values and standards have changed over time, and realise you are putting up today with behaviour that a few years ago you would have believed unthinkable.

Is your child stealing from you? Is your child staying in bed till mid-afternoon? Is he or she constantly throwing temper tantrums? Throwing furniture about? Coming in at all hours? Threatening you? Blackmailing you? Your self-esteem is probably in your boots right now, but however you regard yourself as a parent, good or bad or sometimes both, it doesn't set aside that one basic, unalterable truth, *you do not have to accept unacceptable behaviour.*

Just because you're a parent, you do not have to put up with anything and everything your youngster likes to chuck at you. You, too, have rights – and one of them is enjoyment of a quiet life at home. Think about it.

Are you doing them a favour – or are you in fact, silently condoning their anti-social behaviour? How are they to know what you really mean if you do not back up your words with actions? As we saw earlier, it is actions which express intentions and meanings. If you *say*, 'I don't want you to do such and such,' but you continue to allow them to do 'such and such' in your home, you are in fact giving them permission to carry right on. You are saying, *by your own behaviour*, that doing 'such and such' is OK by you.

If your child is also a person, think about what you would do if it were a distant relative who had invaded your home and was behaving like this? What would you think? What would you do?

Jennet, a single parent with a troubled sixteen year old, was very frightened of him. She had banned from her home a youth called Johnny, whom she guessed was a dealer, but one day her son Peter brought Johnny home. There was a confrontation between Jennet and her son. He refused to send Johnny away and Johnny refused to go. 'This is my home and I can invite anyone I like here,' said Peter. At her wits' end Jennet said, 'Well I shall go for the police.'

Before they could stop her she slipped out of the house and went to the local police, asking them for help. She explained the situation, that she was alone with her son, that there was a drugs dealer in the house and she needed someone to 'make it stick'. Two officers came back with her. As she had expected (and as she had warned the police), there was no sign of Johnny and the windows of her son's room were wide open, to air the room and get rid of any evidence.

56

The police towered over Peter and told him a few pithy truths – not least the fact that 'if your mother says she doesn't want someone here, they don't come here, if your mother says "jump", you jump, if your mother says "out" you're out. And don't let us have to come here again or you'll really regret it'. The whole operation lasted ten minutes.

After they had gone, Peter sat with his head in his hands for about half an hour. He was stunned that his mother had actually got the police into the house, that she had shopped him herself and even risked prosecution – since if evidence of drugs had been found there, technically she would have been responsible.

It need hardly be said that Peter did not repeat the behaviour. He sulked at first, but he became very careful about how he behaved with his mother. This was the first of a number of positive actions Jennet took which ultimately led him to ask for help. Peter has been off drugs for over a year now.

It is not suggested that you may necessarily need to go to the lengths Jennet did. Every situation is different. The important thing is to recognise that inside you is a great well of inner strength – your own right *to be*.

By working on yourself, by building up your own self-respect and your shattered sense of self-worth, you will gradually recover your own equilibrium and begin to tap your positive, healthy source of parent-power. The aim of this whole exercise is very straightforward:

It is to make you believe in yourself again – and to enable you to create a situation in which your troubled teenager no longer finds it convenient, comfortable or even possible to 'misbehave'.

You are going to get the strength to work creatively so that you do not stand in the way of your child reaching out for help. By your own actions, or *lack of action*, you can take positive steps towards saving your child's life or sanity.

Your Painful Emotions

We will now look at some of the emotions we have discussed earlier. Think about those which you recognise in yourself:

Fear. Anger/Resentment. Guilt/Self-Blame. Shame. Envy/ Jealousy. Suspiciousness. Loneliness/Isolation. Self Pity/ Despair. Depression.

Not a pretty lot, are they? They are hard to live with, and they don't exactly make you easy for other people to live with either. It isn't only you who suffers from these emotions. Everybody gets the backlash – your partner (who is probably suffering similarly), the rest of your family and any close friends or relatives you may have. In your heart you know this to be true and that only lowers your sense of self-worth. The vicious circle is set up.

What we are going to do is look at ways of breaking that vicious circle of painful emotions, so that you recover your self-esteem.

Fear

Fear comes in many forms. The most extreme fear a parent can have is that their child may die, or suffer grave physical or mental damage. There is also the fear of prison and lesser, but very real fears that your child may just end up on the scrap heap, with no qualifications, no training or experience – and no will to make a place for themselves in the sun.

The important thing right now is for you to realise you are not alone. Thousands of other parents are suffering fear like yours – but many others have found ways of overcoming it and you can too. Right now you may be too rigid with terror to believe it, but it is true.

Even if the worst has seemed to have happened and your child is mainlining on heroin or out of his or her mind on butane or glue, there is still hope. Just concentrate on the fact that your child is still alive today and that you are now doing something positive and constructive about making the situation better.

For Anne, the worst fears were her nightly vigils outside her daughter's room where she stood listening, trying to hear if her daughter, a heroin addict, was still breathing.

For Jack and Hazel, it was finding Tom lying in the blood spattered bathroom, a syringe across his arm. The dreadful wait for the ambulance, the hours in the hospital waiting room until they were told their boy would live after all.

But Tom, and Anne's daughter, are both alive, and recovering today.

Properly speaking, most fear is concerned with something that hasn't happened yet. The feeling of fear is *now*, but the event that the fear has hooked to has not yet arrived. You do not fear anything that has happened in the past. You may feel sad or angry or depressed because of it, but you do not fear it. You may fear that something from the past may happen again. It is the future recurrence of the event you fear. In other words fear is always connected with the future. Anne, Jack and Hazel all feared their children were going to die.

But you live *now*. You cannot live in the future. You cannot write a future script for events, rehearse a future conversation, foresee a future action. The future always springs surprises. You cannot live your child's life for tomorrow, nor even your own. You can only cope with events that are happening to you now, today. And today you are alive and so is your troubled child. For today that is enough. Today you are finding out about a way to cope which you didn't have yesterday. Today things begin to get better.

The most practical way of dealing with fear is to start, right now, living in today. Do not consider tomorrow. You can make general plans, of course. But hang on to the thought that just for today you can handle whatever is dished out to you. And you can, you know. You do not disintegrate because of what happens today.

If, like millions of people who never or hardly ever go near a church or a synagogue or any other such place, you have a sneaking belief in any Greater or Inner Power, start putting it to work for you, in your everyday life. If you can, take a leap of faith. Someone remarked that she'd never heard of anyone who didn't arrive on dry land after taking that leap. When things get tough, just pause a minute. Keep a still silence inside you. You may be surprised at what happens.

Guilt and Self-Blame

The generalised guilt which society shoves on parents is useless baggage. To be sure, in small ways, sometimes in large, we have behaved badly to our children, but breastbeating and carrying a load of unspecified guilt is not going to help either them or you now. So accept, first of all, that you love your child even though that child behaves sometimes so horribly that you hate them. The opposite of love is not hate, but indifference. If you are so battered and scarred today that you do feel indifferent, don't worry. When things start to get better your real feelings will come back and you'll be able to love again.

The next way to get rid of guilt is to accept that you are not God. If your son or daughter is going to use dangerous or illegal drugs, if they intend to drink to excess, if they persist in promiscuous sex, gamble excessively or refuse to eat, there is no practical way you can stop them.

You can talk, threaten, lock them in, turn away their friends, stop their pocket money, beat them, weep at them, describe in graphic detail the horrors of addiction or prostitution – but *you cannot control them*. If a person of any age decides to abuse substances, alcohol, sex or fruit machines, that person will do so, if not today, then tomorrow or next week.

Unless you envisage a life entirely given over to becoming a jailer, you would be wise to accept that energy spent in trying to control another person's actions, is energy wasted. That applies even if the person is very young indeed – your dearly loved child. There are plenty of things that you can do which will radically alter the situation but preventing someone from taking drink, drugs or gambling is not among them. There are constructive ways to use that energy.

Also, whatever anyone may say, your child's drugging, drinking or gambling *is not your fault.* You may think yourself a pretty imperfect parent, but everyone, even a small child, knows what is dangerous, illegal and perhaps lethal. If a teenager chooses to act in these ways that choice has been theirs, *not* yours.

Guilt works in devious ways. When a youngster gets into trouble, all too often a parent will take on full responsibility. 'Where did I go wrong? ... if only I hadn't sent them to that school ... been stricter ... less strict .. stopped the kid going to discos ... hadn't had so many children ... had a brother or sister for them.' I have known a desperate mother guiltily reviewing her whole life, blaming herself for every event she could remember happening to her addict son, even going back in time to blame herself for being his mother. Guilt leads to a kind of self-destructive madness.

As has been said, tiresome teenagers are a commonplace in every household. It is sad but true that teenagers in deep trouble are not uncommon in many households today. Cocaine and heroin were once the sole property of the rich. In the sixties and early seventies, cannabis and LSD were a middle class problem. Now they are all available in housing estates, school playgrounds up and down the country, relatively cheaply, together with an infinite number of other mind and mood altering substances.

Part of the process of being a teenager is belonging to a group of friends, whose influence is, for a time, in some ways greater than the influence of home. If just one member of the group starts a fashion that it is 'cool' to use this or that substance, then there's a chance that many of the group will follow. What happens after that – whether a youngster continues to use that substance, graduates to others, or decides to leave it alone depends on an enormous number of factors. What goes on at home is only one of them. If your child is one of those hundreds of thousands who 'use', then it is essential to accept that you didn't cause it – but you can find ways to cope with it.

Guilt is unproductive. It was your child's destiny to be born into your family at just the time and place it happened. You cannot change that. What you can change is what you do about it now.

Earlier we discussed society's readiness to cast blame on parents. Well, anybody can *cast* blame, but you don't need to accept it – whether the person who does the casting is your child, a teacher, psychiatrist, social worker, probation officer or whoever. Just hang on to the fact that you are *not* guilty.

The last thing you ever wanted was for your kid to get into trouble, right? So remember you are merely one among many influences in your child's life. There are many others: your partner (if any), brothers and sisters, neighbours, aunts, uncles, schoolfriends – and, heaven help us, the media – to name but a few. All these have affected the way your child sees and reacts to the world. You may often have been mistaken, but you have tried to do what you thought was best. Unfortunately you were not God and it didn't turn out the way you wanted. Tough. But things can get better, as you will find out, if you are willing to make the effort. Start to forgive yourself today.

If your child truly decided to change his or her behaviour, you would forgive the past, wouldn't you? Then do the same for yourself.

Anger and Resentment

Of course you are angry. It's perfectly normal. When your house and home has been thrown into chaos by a troubled teenager, if you didn't feel angry you wouldn't be human.

So accept it. Don't sit in judgement on your feelings. Don't bottle them up. They'll only come out at unexpected and inappropriate times. You'll blow your stack over something quite trivial or get deeply depressed and end up by not functioning at all.

You are probably angry at: your child, dealers and the whole drug industry, publicans and owners of the fruit machine alleys. You are angry with the law for letting these things happen. At your child's friends, especially the person who you think 'led them into all this trouble'. You may also be angry about their school, their work (or lack of it), at the government or the whole rotten world. Finally, and most importantly, you are angry with yourself (or your partner) for not having stopped it happening.

Most of us are brought up to believe that anger is an unacceptable emotion. We pretend it doesn't exist and try to cover it up. But anger is a very useful and important emotion which does not have to lead to destruction. It can also be a goad to make things better. If Wilberforce hadn't been angry about the rottenness of slavery, slaves would have been in chains that much longer.

So accept your anger. You can't help having emotions, anyway, so take a good long look at your anger. Write down all the things you are angry about. Every irritation and resentment large and small. Get it all down on paper. Just doing that will clear your mind a bit.

Now let's look at where we are. Right now you are in the middle of confusion. There's not much chance of doing anything immediately effective about the law, the government, the state of society or the world. Perhaps later you can start a crusade, but right now you have more pressing problems – namely to get your own house in order.

So we'll start where the trouble seems to begin: with your child. If you accept that your child is suffering from an illness, then you have only one option. You love the child and hate the illness. Your anger is about the illness, not about the person. A youngster suffering from addiction can no more stop telling lies and stealing than a person with cerebral palsy can stop shaking. The only difference between addiction and cerebral palsy is that the illness of addiction can be arrested. Addicts *can* recover.

Your anger is normal when your child breaks the furniture, steals, lies, overdoses, injects lethal substances. Partly it is caused by sheer terror.

When I say accept your anger, I mean accept that you feel the way you do. When I say you have no control over your emotions, I mean that it is proper to feel angry when unacceptable things happen to you or your home or other members of the family. But – and this is vital – you do have control about what you do about your anger. You do have control about how you express it. Throwing a temper-tantrum, bullying, shouting, screaming, hitting people – these are *not* acceptable or adult ways of expressing your anger.

It can be hard to learn new ways of behaving, but the dividends are immense. At the beginning we all fail lots of times, but if you stick at it, it gets easier and the whole atmosphere begins to change.

Some ways to deal with your anger:

1. Write it all down, read it through and then burn it, or share it with a close friend.
2. Talk it all out with a friend who understands the situation.
3. Go and dig the garden, furiously beat a pillow, or find an open place and scream your head off (I leave it to you to decide what you say with every spadeful of earth, every thump on the pillow or every word of that scream!)
4. Talk to your child (if that is where your anger is directed) and explain that you feel anger. This is where you tread very carefully. Keep it simple. It will be enough to say 'I want to tell you that I am very angry because you lied to me today.' Do not refer to all the other times your child has lied to you, do not refer to all the good things you have showered on them in the past. Do not harp on how they have failed you time and time again. They know it all too well.

If you are feeling great surges of anger about a dealer or somebody who you believe 'led' your youngster into his troubled waters, then you are not unusual, because most parents in your position feel the same. But like so many of our negative feelings, it is useless baggage. Your anger over this merely eats *you* up – and leaves the other untouched. It is very salutary to consider the probable behaviour of your own youngster. If he or she is in the drink, drugs or gambling whirlpool it is almost certain that they have also been responsible for leading someone else into it. As far as drugs are concerned, unless your youngster has a private income, then there are only three ways of supporting any habit – whether it's marijuana or heroin.

64

Stealing, dealing or prostitution. With some drugtakers, it's more a matter of 'sharing' than 'dealing', but it certainly means drawing newcomers into the charmed circle. So before you start brooding over the evils which X or Y has done to your child, consider those other parents who have every reason to believe the same about yours. It's sad but, alas, true.

When Your Child is Angry With You

Troubled children spill out anger like lava from an erupting volcano. It spews over everyone, whether it's expressed in shouting, in silence, in apathy or in physical destruction.

The anger of a sick, addicted child is anger with him or herself. Addicts know they are destroying themselves, but they are unable (just at the moment) to stop. They hate themselves, and they use their nearest and dearest as whipping boards. When this happens, when your child's anger erupts, just keep remembering that the anger is in him or her. Do not allow yourself to be sucked into it.

There is a very effective technique for dealing with this. Just imagine there is a mirror between you and your child. Visualise him or her shouting obscenities (they very often are obscenities) back at themselves because deep down that's what they really are doing. Detach yourself from the whole thing. They're sick. Simply walk away from it, in your mind, or in person, if you can. They may come ranting and raving after you, towering over you, shouting words of hate and anger, but just get on with what you're doing. If there's a pause, you can say in a conversational way, 'I'm making some coffee. Would you like a cup?' or 'I'm just going to telephone your grandfather. Do you want to talk to him?' or whatever you like. But see that it is quite matter of fact and entirely unrelated to the nonsense.

Having a tirade ignored as if they were mentally defective (or you were deaf) is very deflating. When your child has kept you in a web of terror and anger for months or even years, it is very unsettling to find their fury falling upon unresponsive ears. It makes them think, which is exactly what you want them to do. It may be hard – and the first few times you might not be too successful – but with practice, it becomes a mighty powerful tool. Practise.

The Core of Your Own Anger

Over time, by handling your day-to-day anger in the ways that have been suggested above, you will find that you are recognising it more quickly, and getting more able to deal with it, before it explodes inside you.

If you really want to grow and be less at the mercy of your anger, you will need to go beyond the first-aid steps suggested here and get to know yourself a great deal more deeply.

There is not the time and space for it in this book, but in brief I can tell you that *your* anger is also your own. It is not caused and created by anything or anybody outside yourself, but it has appeared because you have allowed yourself to become angry. Your anger is *yours*, just as much as your troubled child's anger belongs to him or her.

To find out where your anger springs from takes time, thought and often a great deal of painful self-searching. It means tracing your feelings back to the earliest times you experienced them. It means 'owning' them. It means coming to terms with the first occasions for anger and the people to whom you were close in your early life (your parents, sisters, brothers and so on) – and then forgiving them. It means also ultimately forgiving yourself.

In the last analysis all destructive emotions can be traced back to guilt, fear and anger. These three are the springs of all unhappiness and pain in yourself – and all, in time, can be recognised and knocked out of action with the tools suggested in this book.

Shame Leading to Isolation

Shame just doesn't apply. If your child is suffering from an addiction, your child is ill. Addiction is no less an illness than diabetes or cancer. Would you feel shame if your child suffered from these? This is not to say that some of the behaviour may not be socially embarrassing, but remember, the behaviour is a symptom of the illness. An epileptic fit in a supermarket may also be embarrassing, but it is no cause for shame.

Mary and James are well known citizens in their local community. Their daughter Sara figured largely in the local paper on a shoplifting charge (getting money for her addiction). But Mary and James knew their daughter was ill – not evil – and continued to hold their heads high, even managing to live sanely in the chaos created by the troubled daughter. Over time, as they put into their lives many of the suggestions in this book, friends would come to see them amazed, 'How can you look so well with all the trouble you've got?' They can, because they have dealt with shame the only practical way in these circumstances. As Mary put it:

1. She has accepted that she has no control over anyone else's life but her own.
2. She has accepted that addiction is an illness, not a moral sin.
3. She has given her daughter directions about where to get help.
4. She has released her daughter – with love – to make her own decisions.
5. She has learnt to live her own life, not her daughter's.

It should not surprise you to learn that Sara is drug-free today and has not had a drink or drug for several months.

Envy and Jealousy Leading to Isolation

Ruth, a divorced mother, has three children. All three of them showed serious signs of drugs misuse. She admitted to being full of envy for other parents whose children appeared to have no problems. She was consumed with shame every time a friend asked her about her children. She began avoiding people – crossing the road if an acquaintance appeared. She stopped telephoning friends and invited nobody home, thus increasing her sense of isolation and loneliness.

She had no partner to share the responsibility with her. Her ex-husband, smarting because she had divored him, blamed her for their children's addiction – and she accepted this blame. Her only brother, much older, lived in another city, and they weren't close. But her brother's two children were straight, successful and high achievers. She was filled with shame, envy and self-pity whenever she thought about her brother and his children. 'Why me?' was her constant cry.

Like guilt, envy and jealousy bring no profit. The only person who suffers from your envy is yourself. The people you envy go merrily on their way unimpaired and unhurt by your envious feelings. Only you are hurt and paralysed into inaction if you allow the bitterness to engulf you. So it is with all of us.

There are always people better off than oneself but also people worse off. Perhaps – like Ruth – you believe there is nobody with such an appalling set of problems as yours.

But Ruth found, not long after she had joined Families Anonymous, that there were indeed others worse off than herself. She met a bewildered and devastated couple all of whose four children were heroin addicts. She met a mother and father who had suffered the death of one of their five children through drugs and now had another child who was a heroin addict. At least Ruth's three were still alive.

Life doesn't dish out all the bad things simultaneously to everyone. But it does seem to have a way of evening out the score. Over time, everyone gets their ration of pain, grief, joy and delight. That family you so envy today, with their happy successful children all succeeding and 'straight' may be destined to all manner of unforseen calamities tomorrow.

Indeed, unknown to you they may have suffered before, or be suffering today, and you do not know of it. There are a hundred pains and agonies which are endured behind closed doors. Not everyone's problems are manifested in a drunken child lurching into the house at midnight.

Ways to squash envy:

1. Find some people in a similar or worse plight to yourself and see what you can do to get close to them. Perhaps you can

share some of your suffering with them, and together ease each other's pain. (In the back of this book there is a list of organisations which are self-help groups and which offer boundless opportunities for this).

2. Go back to the basics and start with the good things that you have. Have you had food today? Have you a roof over your head? Clothes? Carpet? A telephone? Legs? Arms? Eyes to see with? I know this may sound something like your grandmother might have said but grandmother knew a thing or two. It works. It really works. In moments of great pain, many people (including me) have used this method of getting a sense of perspective. 'This too will pass' is something to hang on to.

3. Start believing, today, that your child will recover. You are doing all you can. Many, many addicts recover. Yours can too. Have faith. Two of Ruth's three children are well and straight today.

Rights and Privileges – which are whose?

Troubled, troublesome youngsters have a quite remarkable capacity for explaining their rights. They have a 'right' to be fed, watered, given bed, board, lodging, spending money, clothes, washing, ironing, telephone service, music, entertainment, leisure. You name it, they've got a right to it. Or so they would have you believe.

There is one right they do not claim – and which you really do owe them. That is the right to learn by their own mistakes. This is probably the only real gift you can make to a teenager in trouble. You can give them the opportunity to experience the consequences of their own decisions.

For many parents this is the gift that it is really hard to give, yet paradoxically, it is the only one which matters.

The child in trouble has refused to heed warnings. Everyone knows there is danger in drugs, that frequenting pubs and gambling joints is likely to lead to trouble. But the pressure from friends, the thrill of risk, the urge to taste forbidden fruit, all these can be more heady and exciting than doom-laden advice from boring old parents who've forgotten what it was like to be young.

So now there's a real problem. Maybe it's bad debts or stolen goods. Perhaps it's a drugs' bust or a charge for drunkenness. Maybe there's trouble at school or social security fraud. Maybe it's just that you, the parent, has found out the truth. This is where it gets not only tough for the youngster, but tough for the parent too.

Your natural instinct to protect your young is reinforced by all sorts of other social considerations: other people finding out, your family reputation down the drain, school career or job being jeopardised, a police record or even a prison sentence. The first time serious trouble arises, most parents' immediate response is to jump in there and bail them out fast.

In reality this may be the most unhelpful thing you can do.

The first appearance before a court has saved more than one very young kid from pursuing further forbidden delights. The price for risk-taking can be found to be too high when confronted with the full panoply of law and order.

There are many ways in which parents can bail children out of unpleasant consequences – giving them sick notes for school when it's clear they are not ill, paying debts to relatives or friends, paying court fines, telephoning employers for them – all sorts of excuses, and not one good reason.

Most parents of addicted youngsters have done most of these things and found that it got them precisely nowhere. Promises to reform are not kept. Loans are not repaid. If you're in the situation you will know the rest. The list is pretty extensive.

As soon as you feel enough strength to carry it through, decide what you really know to be best and do it. If you've been working on your self-respect and getting shot of some of your guilt and self-blame, it will gradually become clear what you can actually manage to handle – for everyone's sake.

When you have begun to put these suggestions into your daily life, you will discover that you know, intuitively, exactly the right moment to tell your youngster where to get help. You will know what rules you can make stick. You will find in yourself the strength to carry out even your toughest ultimatum, because you will know that it is the most loving thing you can do. Susanne's 18 year old son Chris was an alcoholic and an addict. She had told him she would not tolerate certain behaviour in her home, especially stealing. He stole one more time. Although he was two stone underweight, had nowhere to go except to druggy friends, had no money, no skill and no will to work, she told him to leave home. Within a week he'd been thrown out of the squat he went to, and found his way to an Alcoholics Anonymous meeting. Sometime earlier, Susanne had told him where to get help for himself. When the chips were down and he had nowhere left to go he took the step which was to lead to his recovery. He had reached his 'rock bottom'.

Love has dimensions of justice and responsibility. Love is not just indiscriminate giving and forgiving. Parent-power is about allowing those you love to take responsibility for their own lives and especially for their own mistakes. This is their right – and the most loving gift you can give them.

Marriage Under Stress

As we have observed, troubled teenagers have a gift for manipulation. Nowhere is this more evident than in their capacity for setting parents against each other. It is quite easy really. Usually one parent is a softer touch than the other. With some smart footwork and the iron determination which springs from compulsive need, parents can be divided and ruled.

A family with a seriously troubled child is almost certainly an unhealthy family. And the strains this illness puts upon marriage cannot be exaggerated.

First there is the clear manipulation ('Daddy says I *can* have the car') and the subterfuge ('Don't tell your father I'm giving you this'), but finally the truth will have to be faced.

This is when the blame starts flying – bouncing like a poltergeist round the whole house. 'If you hadn't been so hard on him' ... 'If you hadn't brought her up to be a Jewish princess' ... 'If you'd sent him to the other school' ... 'If it wasn't for the way your mother spoilt her rotten' ... 'If you'd only spent more time with him when he was little – like taking him fishing' ... 'If you didn't drink so much' ... 'If only you'd given her half the attention you gave her brother' ... all the old scabs and sores that haven't been properly dealt with are picked raw and bleeding. The theme is, 'It's all your fault'. In fact, although sometimes neither will admit it, each parent feels it is 'all my fault'.

This is exactly the situation which most suits the troubled child. As long as the parents are fighting it out, there is a good chance that the child can walk into the battlefield and pick up all the loot while the contenders are still crossing swords.

Insane, isn't it? When I say, health begins with one person and spreads outwards, this is true. But if *both* parents agree on what is acceptable behaviour, if both, together, decide how to act towards their afflicted child, then the chance of the child asking for help is more than doubled. And that's what you both want, isn't it?

So drop the cudgels and start looking inwards. Accept that you are powerless over your child's life – and that of your partner. Accept that you have a lot of pent-up anguish, anger, fear, guilt, shame and frustration. But accept that you can have power over your own actions and your own reactions.

'*Your* faults are so glaringly obvious, and well, I suppose I have a few faults too – but mostly they were caused by you anyway.' Or, 'I was just a bit thoughtless. Everyone's thoughtless sometimes. You can't expect me to be perfect'. It's a great deal easier to point out the other person's faults than to take steps to identify and deal with your own.

Tell your partner honestly what you know to be necessary for your own self-respect and peace of mind. Listen to your partner in silence and with an open mind. No one is wholly right or wholly wrong. It's not much good setting rules that one or other of you just cannot stick to. Sort out your own priorities – together – and not in front of your child. It's not as easy to do as to say, but it's possible if you both really want all the family to get well.

The Special Predicament of Fathers

Much as I dislike sexist distinctions, it has to be said that many fathers find it hard to acknowledge the existence of a 'problem' in a child. When forced to confront it, they frequently suffer the added stress of not being able to talk about it. The inhuman assumption that men should endure without complaint or tears the most bitter anguish, pain and guilt takes a huge toll. All too many men have been bred to believe that when trouble occurs they must arise and *act*.

The action may take the form of heavy-handed homilies, heavy-handed beltings, or heavy-handed use of the drinks cabinet. Alternatively it may be making good the debts, accepting the promises of your about-to-reform son or daughter (and giving them a golden handshake to seal the bargain), or sitting down to give them a rational explanation of the harm s/he is doing to his or her career, life, future prospects and so on. The most drastic action of either parent may be throwing your child into the street with no indication that there can be a way out.

All the fathers I have spoken to have reacted in one or other of these ways, initially. And that word *react* is the heart of the matter. 'Action' is another thing altogether. It may involve non-action. But action is positive, reaction is not only negative, it can prolong your child's agony, and your own.

Non-action in such ways as refusing to pay bad debts is actually very strong action indeed. Non-action in refusing to give money however heavy the blackmail ('I'll have to steal it then') is very powerful stuff. It means you are prepared to stand up for what you believe. And paying off pushers, dealers, overdrafts, loans and the like is not something you surely believe is right? If you already have reacted by throwing your child out, there's a strong chance you won't have seen the last of them. Sometime or another they will certainly be in touch with someone in the family, even if they are seething with resentment against you personally. Don't worry. You can still get word that there *is* hope and that you'll help when they really mean business.

73

The frustration which afflicts the fathers of youngsters in trouble is terrible. The combination of fear for their lives and deeply wounded pride can be devastating. It is almost inconceivable that your child can choose a life-style which should more properly be called a death-style. It is beyond comprehension that you are powerless to convince that child of the hideous error of their ways. Yet until your powerlessness over anyone else's compulsion is recognised and acknowledged, you will continue to wage a losing war. If your child chooses death, insanity or prison – then you must accept and respect their decision. Without guilt and without self blame.

Easy to say. Not so easy to do. But some of the tools for this exercise are outlined in this book. You may be surprised how effective they are, if you work at them. Admission of your own frailty and powerlessness oddly confers unexpected power.

Two fathers were talking about their children's addiction problems. 'I'm a rational man,' said one. 'I just could not understand how James could possibly want to continue with his habit when he saw what harm he was doing to himself, and all of us.' 'I didn't either,' said the other father, 'until Alistair put it to me straight. He told me one day that he did not want anything else but heroin. That made sense. If that *was* the only thing he wanted, then his behaviour had a kind of rationality. It helped me come to terms with it'. Coming to terms with a great many unpalatable facts is what all this is about.

Sisters and Brothers

There are three ways in which brothers and sisters can be damaged by a family member suffering from one of the addictions. The first is obvious. They can be lured into the scene, either because the addict is older and it looks glamorous, or because the addict is younger and the older one feels responsible and wants to keep an 'eye on the kid'. Either way, they play the addict's game.

Secondly, they can be let into the guilty secret and pressured to keep it from the parents. I have talked with numbers of brothers and sisters who had taken on this role. One girl knew for three years that her brother was abusing heroin but had managed to carry this fearful burden without guidance or support, trying desperately to help him in her own way and, at the same time, to cover up for him whenever there was danger of the parents' finding out. She was later to admit that she became as crazy, as devious, dishonest and as guilt-ridden as her brother. Her own life became secondary. She felt a failure because she could do nothing to stop him – but her world revolved around him and his sick activities.

The third way in which brothers and sisters are affected is by neglect. A family with a child suspected of addiction, particularly to drink or to drugs, centres round that child. Sisters and brothers usually get short shrift. Their proper concerns are brushed aside. Time and again I have heard parents say how guilty they have felt because they gave so little attention to the rest of the family – whether they were having successes or failures – because the addict demanded (and got) all the attention.

Brothers and sisters can be left with a bitter legacy of anxiety, guilt and envy. There may be compassion, but there will certainly be anger whether it is acknowledged or not. In a family dominated by addiction, most of these emotions are inappropriately expressed or unhealthily denied.

But the same principle of recovery applies to brothers and sisters as applies to parents. You can't save anybody's life but your own. Quite literally you are not your brother's keeper, nor your sister's. You cannot cover up for ever. You don't have to fall for blackmail. The longer you cover up, the longer they suffer.

If you feel neglected, you probably are. But there are things you can do about it. You can get in touch with one of the organisations listed in the back of this book. Or if that's not for you, just keep reading and try especially to work on your own sense of self-respect and self-esteem. While the whole family is sick (including you I'm sorry to say) there's no help in wallowing in a soggy mass of self-pity. You can start by cleaning up your own act. When you can be sure that you're doing the right things for yourself, you'll be less dependent on others for approval. That alone is a big step towards the maturity which so many of us claim, but so few of us really have – however many years we may have under the belt.

A Family Sickness

What do we really want our children to be like? I imagine most of us would want to see them getting on well in their own lives, being courteous and considerate around the house, being cheerful and happy. We'd like them to be good-tempered and self-disciplined. We'd like them to have plenty of self-respect but to be able to apologise and admit it when they are wrong. Above all, we'd want them to be courageous and honest.

The trouble with living with other people is that we all act and react on each other. And when one member of the family gets emotionally ill, it can creep up gradually until the whole family begins to act and react in unhealthy ways, often without anyone even realising it until real disaster looms.

This is particularly so when the trouble is addiction or related behaviour. Personality profiles of the family members taken in tests at one illustrious medical treatment centre for alcoholism and addiction have established that the families of patients show 'gross personality disorders'. In some cases, these are even more serious than those of the patient.

Makes you think, doesn't it?

For this reason, if for no other, the next section is very important indeed. If your child is sick, there's quite a chance that you, too, are in need of help. What you will find outlined in the following pages are some clear directions for self-help. It is easy to read but don't imagine it's going to be easy to put into practice in your everyday living. It isn't. On the other hand you can be certain of one thing. When you begin to put these ideas and principles into your day-to-day living, everything will start to get better.

As far as your child is concerned, it won't look like that at all. But bear in mind, what you are aiming for is that 'rock-bottom' – that moment of truth. If your child reacts badly at the beginning – even appears to be getting worse – you're in there with a chance. Parent-power is beginning to work.

Listen to that recovered heroin addict, Sara. 'When my parents told me I could get on with my own life and they were going to stop worrying about me I thought, "Great – I can get stoned whenever I like now." But a couple of weeks later they stopped my pocket money and I even had to take sandwiches to school. One thing led to another – they took away all my props so I really had no choice left except to ask for treatment. Thank God they stopped "enabling" me.'

So we start, not with the children but with you – the parents. All those splendid characteristics you'd like your children to have – how many of them are you currently displaying? If you are bedevilled by a troubled and troublesome teenager there is a fair chance that you are displaying very few of them. Oddly enough, the most important is:

Getting On With Life – Your Own Life

When you are frantic with worry, desperate for help for your child, uncertain about what to do for the best, every waking moment seems to be spent thinking about how to get them straightened out. You lie awake at night, fearful and anxious, trying to figure out ways of making them change or rehashing your own past errors.

In other words, you are living a life through your troubled or addicted child. If you look at it squarely you are just as addicted as your child. Your child may be spending all their waking hours thinking about the next drink, drug, gamble or fix and you are doing the same about him or her. It is no good. You might even manage to get the kid sent abroad or away – but they'll take themselves with them – and the problem is in themselves.

What is even worse, your own life is dripping away and you are slipping into what is actually a family sickness. Probably you are ignoring the very real concerns of the rest of the family. You are always walking on eggshells. All conversation comes back to the 'problem' of Johnny, or Susan, or whoever is your troubled child. Nobody else gets any of your attention – least of all yourself.

Face this fact – you cannot help anyone if you are in pieces. So the first job you have to do is start by putting your *own* life together.

It can be a very tough job, especially for mothers who have been conditioned to sacrifice themselves for their children through thick and thin. There are, however, good, concrete reasons why you should get your own life in shape:

a) Kids in trouble suffer enormous problems of guilt. If they see you anguished and distressed about them, it gives them yet another reason for not facing their own problem – and gives them yet another reason to drink, gamble or drug. It won't show as guilt. It will probably come out in anger, but guilt it is. Letting them see how seriously they have damaged you and your life is doing them no favour. It just piles on the guilt.

b) If you are doing the worrying for them, why should they worry? If you are tidying up the messes in their life, whether it's telling lies about them to the police or pretending they haven't actually stolen any money from you, if *you* are taking responsibility for their lives and actions, why should they bother? You are stopping them from growing up.

c) You have a duty and a right to your own life. It's all you've got. You probably slid into this spiral of unhealthy despair through the sickness of your child. So if *you* get well, good health will spread back to your child. Sickness is contagious but so is health. Just try and you will find out.

Self-Respect

The worst thing about lack of self-respect is that it is self-perpetuating. The more badly you feel yourself treated, the more it will happen. If you feel ripped off, taken for a ride, used up, pillaged, put upon and you aren't doing anything about it, then it will go on occurring.

If you've got into the way, like so many mothers (and some

78

fathers) of 'putting the children first', doing everything for them, putting your own needs last (if at all), then for everyone's sake, you are going to have to start thinking about your own needs. Many mothers have almost forgotten they have any needs. The endless round of working and serving other people's requirements and wants has often bereft them of a knowledge of what they do need to feel good in themselves. By that I do *not* mean feeling good because your partner has been promoted at work, or your son has got a good school report. All too many mothers accept fulfilment through other people's sucesses and achievements.

What I am talking about is finding out what makes *you* yourself feel good. Oddly enough, one of the most miraculous ways of making yourself feel good is saying 'NO'!

You are hoping that one day your troubled child will be able to say 'no' to whatever is troubling them? Well, the first step for you to do is to learn to say 'NO' and make it stick. The first time you do this you will probably be rather alarmed. You will fall back into the pattern of wondering whether your refusal to do whatever your child wants, will make them do something terrible, or become violent or threatening or, worst of all, stop loving you. Right?

Let's take an example. Eddie has asked you for more money. You know he wants it for drugs. 'Only a loan, Mum, I promise to pay it back.' Your old pattern was to nag and ask the reason and go on about broken promises and then finally to 'lend' him the money, for fear if you didn't give it to him, he would steal it or do something worse. Now you have to dare to say 'NO' – and mean it. You don't have to give any reasons. It is your own decision. Just plain 'NO'.

You probably will get a tirade or some heavy emotional blackmail. Ignore it. Pretend you aren't hearing it. Get on with whatever you are doing and if there's a pause, say something quite pleasant in a quiet conversational voice. Something like, 'I'm just going to make a cup of tea, would you like one?'

It is vital not to enter into any discussion. It isn't necessary and it won't get you anywhere. Kids know all the answers and they've had years of practice in twisting you round their thumb.

Start giving reasons and you are sunk. The only explanation you need give – if you like – is 'I don't choose to.'

After all, why should you give him money? You wouldn't be saying no if it were his proper, regular pocket money. This is a loan. Well it's *your* money and you can do exactly what you like with it – and what you like is not to 'lend' any to him. Don't say all that. Just say 'NO' and stick to it.

Your kid will probably be surprised. If you're like many other parents with troubled youngsters, you've been so thoroughly manipulated over the months or years, it will come as a nasty shock that you can be so straightforward and blunt. It will be even nastier when they discover that they can't budge you.

But it will be the beginning of self-respect for you, and self-respect is the first and greatest of every human's needs. The importance of saying 'NO' can hardly be exaggerated. A parent of a (now recovering) addict said, 'I never realised how *affirmative* the word "no" really is.'

It is also a relief for your unhappy child. If your child knows you are going to stick to the rules, an element of safety will come back into their life. While they are careering, unbridled and headstrong through the whole family, laying waste and havoc all around, they are at the same time desperate for someone to stop them, to set limits *and stick to them*. By starting with yourself, you begin to help.

Consideration (mainly for mothers)

Yes, this virtue you very likely do have, in large measure. In fact your whole life is probably given over to considering the needs, wishes, wants, desires, demands and requests of the whole family, particularly if you are a mother. If anything, you've probably got a counter-productive amount of consideration for other people.

There's one person, however, that you have probably overlooked, who is gravely in need of mothering. It's yourself.

Now, how, in the name of all that's reasonable, can you expect to be helpful if you're simply a machine for fulfilling other people's needs? *You* are a human being too, remember?

You need consideration. The best favour you can do the whole family is to take care of your own health and needs. Maybe you need an hour's rest in the middle of the afternoon? Maybe you need a day away on your own, walking in a park, reading a book or magazine once a week? For sure you need some time to refuel in some way, to stock up your own internal larder. Have you ever had an urge to paint, to pot, to learn a foreign language, to play an instrument or table-tennis, to skate, to swim? What on earth is stopping you?

Chances are that your partner watches some sport or plays it? Football, golf, fishing, pools, darts, snooker, has a few pints at the pub or plays squash with friends?

But only a very small percentage of women actually 'play'. If they do anything outside the home, it is usually connected with some useful skill, like typing or upholstery which either gives them a way of making money outside the home or saves money within it. Do you do anything just for the sheer fun of it?

One mother, Heather, who had two drug addicted children, kept her sanity by joining a weekly painting class at the evening Adult Institute. She'd never painted before, nobody could say she was likely to push Beryl Cook from her pinnacle, but Heather got great strength from just spending one evening a week doing something just for herself.

It may seem quite a senseless suggestion, when your child is snorting heroin, to propose that you go and start a course in Holiday Spanish. But, believe me, if you start taking care of yourself and getting back your own life and sense of self then, firstly, it will take away some of the guilt your youngster is carrying about, secondly, it will make you a great deal nicer to live with and thirdly you will start getting consideration from the rest of the family.

When you start having some consideration for yourslf, it quite frequently has a domino effect. Others begin to see you more as a person, less as the universal provider of services.

Martyrs may be fine on the walls of a church, but in the general way, they aren't much fun to live with. Martyr-mothers get a kick out of feeling sorry for themselves, enjoy saying how much they do for everyone, how badly treated they are and how much they have to put up with.

What martyr-mothers do not see is that martyrdom is a highly effective way of getting power.

If you are doing things for people, always making them beholden to you, you're powerful, aren't you? People are forever in your debt. The martyr-mother usually doesn't like to be given something in return. Offered a cup of tea in bed, she will say, 'No thanks, I'm so used to getting it myself, I might just as well.' The martyr-mother gets all the pleasure from giving – and never gives anyone else a chance of having that same pleasure. Martyr-mothers never consider themselves – and often declare, 'Nobody has any consideration for me.'

The fact is, people cannot tell by telepathy what your needs are. Many men appear to be conditioned from birth to know, express and usually get their needs fulfilled. But women often do not easily know what their needs are. Oh, everyone knows their own wants, whether it is a new car, a hall carpet or a climbing plant. *Needs* are different. These are personal, individual and really private. Many women think their needs are entirely concerned with other people's lives – their partner's promotion at work, someone passing a music exam, grandmother getting a home help. These are *not* your *own* needs at all.

When you put yourself out just that little too much for someone, when you feel you've done more than enough, with no returns, then 'consideration' has a nasty habit of turning into resentment.

It has never seemed to me odd that the German word 'Gift' means 'poison' in English. Gifts *can* be poisonous, since every gift brings its own requirement for response. One-sided giving inevitably poisons all relationships.

'Consideration' has other darker aspects. If you look at it in another light, you might sometimes see it as 'people-pleasing'. Do you really always want to do the things you do for people? Or is it that you have a fear deep down that if you don't continue to be a doormat, someone is going to stop loving you?

Think about it. You could be surprised what you come up with.

Admitting When One Is In The Wrong

Earlier, I mentioned that pressured parents can easily fall into the habit of behaving as if everything their troubled child did was wrong, and that they are always in the right. Even when an apology is given, it is all too often wiped out by an attack. A fair sample follows:

'All right, I was wrong to accuse you of stealing that silver spoon, but you've stolen so many things, how was I to know?'

'Yes, I did wrong to hit you but you made me mad.'

'I know I shouldn't have lost my temper but you're always upsetting me and I worry about you so much.'

'I was upset and sarcastic. I admit it. But you do keep doing things that get on my nerves.'

'I know I screamed at you in front of your boyfriend, but you don't realise how tired I am with all the work I have to do...'

Have you noticed the little word 'but'? Does it ring a bell?

An apology with a 'but' almost invariably signals an assault on the other person. Is that really an apology? Or is it making use of a chance to have another go at them – prolonging the row, in effect? Do you *need* to keep it up?

Nobody *made* you mad. Nobody *made* you angry. Nobody *made* you tired. You allowed all these things to happen to you. Your anger is your own responsibility, and so is your worry and your fatigue.

When you have begun to look after yourself, to take care of your own needs, you will not allow yourself to be overworked and overstrained. If you are worried about your child, your family or whatever, that is your own responsibility and there's no need to hang the guilt for this on anyone else, least of all the person you most want to help.

Three fifteen year olds were sitting round in Doreen's kitchen one Saturday afternoon drinking cups of tea. She walked in, took one look at her daughter and said, 'Do you have to look like that? Don't you ever wash? For heaven's sake go and brush your hair.' With a look full of daggers, Sandra went out of the room, saying as she went, 'I think you're bloody rude.' There was an embarrassed silence till Sandra came back, her hair brushed. Doreen sat still for a moment, then with some clearing of the throat, she suddenly said, 'You're right Sandra, I was out of order to talk to you like that in front of your friends. I'm sorry everyone.' The kids all brightened up, the tension passed – and Sandra looked surprised. It was quite out of character for her mother to give an unqualified apology.

What's special about parents – unless it is their integrity? We're all human. We all make mistakes. We can afford to be big about the little things, as long as we hang on to our values about the big things. How can we expect others to take responsibility for their own errors and mistakes if we do not take responsibility for our own?

If a troubled child has good reason for saying, 'Every time anything goes wrong at home, I get the blame,' then they have plenty of alibis for taking the next drink, pill or fix or placing the next bet. If the burden of guilt which they bear within is unrelieved, why should they bother? The simple act of admission of being wrong makes you both human together, you and your child. Whatever the appearances and behaviour may suggest, your child is not a monster but a human being who most certainly isn't *always* in the wrong.

When you begin to practise apologising without 'buts', you'll probably find you get a mouthful back. Ignore it. Don't rise to the bait. If they want to carry on the game, let them. In time it gets easier. In time too you may find the rest of the family will notice and begin to do the same. What you are about is cleaning *your own side of the street*. If they want to go on behaving badly, let them. Just make sure you don't get sucked back into the whirlpool. Every time you bite back that 'but' you win yourself a victory.

If you were quite honest about that list of parental misbehaviour, you'll have ticked quite a few, unless you are quite perfect, in which case you won't be needing to read this book.

Suppose you were a fly on the wall in your own home and saw and heard yourself, would you like what you saw?

Most of us wouldn't. But what to do about it? We'll take a couple for starters.

Criticism

The self-fulfilling prophecy tells us that if we expect the worst from people, by constantly criticising and carping, that's exactly what we'll make happen. Most importantly it works in reverse.

In trying to get out of destructive habits, two things help. The first is that by simply becoming aware of our own actions, we can gradually get control over them and secondly it is usually easier to supplant negative actions with positive ones, rather than just trying to stop doing damaging things. If we're looking for something pleasant to say, we have less time to look at the unpleasant things and less enthusiasm for talking about them.

Mary decided that constant criticism was something she really could and needed to do something about. So she set herself to find something to praise every day in her child's behaviour. The first day it was really difficult to think of anything. They sat at table (one of the rare occasions her daughter actually ate at the same time as her parents) and the mother looked at her pale, unhealthy face, her lank, greasy hair, her scruffy clothes. She knew her daughter hadn't been home the night before.

She was bursting to criticise her about her health, her hours, her appearance, her manner. It seemed impossible to find anything to praise. 'Emily dear, you do have such nice table manners,' she finally managed. She felt extremely foolish, but it was a start.

The important thing was to break the habit of criticism and to look for the good. Mary had the grace to admit that Emily said in reply, 'That's the first nice thing you've said to me in weeks.' After all, *we* like to be praised too, don't we? When someone praises our work, we are pleased and try to continue doing it well. Unfortunately with troublesome teenagers, we sometimes get into a spiral of thinking everything about them as written on the debit side of the ledger, and all our own actions as being on the credit side.

Nagging

'How many times have I told you to ...?.' 'If I've told you once, I've told you a dozen times ... .' Boring isn't it? Furthermore I'd be willing to bet large sums that it has got you precisely nowhere.

No, your youngster isn't deaf, forgetful, or stupid. They just don't want to do it. There can be several reasons for this. The first most innocuous one is that they simply want to show their independence, show they're not 'children' any more. It's certainly a pretty odd way to show you aren't a child, to leave your messes all around – but it isn't the making of messes that they're concerned about, it's *doing what the parent says*.

Second, it may be that bit of growing they are doing at the moment, means that all other considerations are swept aside in the latest pop craze, motor bike mania, or whatever. Total concentration on one thing to the exclusion of all else. This isn't deliberate. It's the teenage version of the absent-minded professor. It's tiresome, but it will pass.

But a third rebellion may occur because the kid has switched off. If every time they come in, they are greeted with a string of complaints, they begin to lose heart, and interest, in pleasing you or any other member of the family. 'Late again ... do you *have* to look so untidy? Pick up your things ... don't leave them there for me to pick up ... you promised to clean your room ... you were late again last night ... I see you came back with that ... do you have to leave crumbs all over the floor ... put out that fag when you speak ... go and wash your hands – and leave the basin clean.' On and on and on!

Would *you* want to please someone who nagged on like that every time you were in a room with them? Wouldn't *you* switch off and think about something else?

Here you have to put in a bit of work. You have to decide what is worth the trouble. What is important. Neither I nor anyone else can tell you how to run your home. You have to decide for yourself whether it's important to you that the washing up is done, whether your son or daughter keeps their rooms tidy, whether it is important to *you* that they do their homework (we'll come back to things like homework later), whether your child appears at meals on time and with clean hands and brushed hair, or just as they are. When you think it through, you can decide what is relatively unimportant and certainly not worth making a fuss over. On the other hand, if you decide something is important to *you*, then make this clear. It's *not* for their own good, but for *yourself* that you require it.

If the response is still negative, you have to decide on action that is reasonably fair, action that you can see through to the end.

Let's take washing up – perhaps the most common irritation. your child dirties stacks of cups and saucers and ashtrays and leaves them all over the house. You can do three things. You can leave them there until green mould grows over the dregs. You can decide that you don't want them all over the house and, *for your own sake*, you can wash them up yourself. Remember, you are doing it to please yourself, because you like a tidy house and lots of clean cups, and you are not expecting any thanks or reward.

You can also do as Edna did. Edna got a bowl, put it on one side of the sink and put all her son's dirty cups and ashtrays into it, telling him that was his washing up, when he wanted to get on with it. The cups were getting short and still the kid didn't wash up his cups (teenagers usually have a very high tolerance of squalor) so Edna took the whole basin of dirties, together with a towel, put the towel on his bed and turned all the cups and saucers and ashtrays onto it. The boy was livid but grudgingly, at last, did his washing up. Edna didn't have to nag about cups any more.

Ways to cope with the compulsion to nag:

1. Get your priorities right. If your child has a serious addiction (drugs, gambling, drinking) leave alone the lesser problems, like smoking, just for the moment.
2. Work out what you can legitimately expect from *any* member of your household and make sure that your troubled

youngster gets a fair share of the work, responsibility and praise.

3. Don't nag about things like school homework or prep. Make sure there is space and time for the child to do it, but be quite clear that whether they do it is *their* problem, not yours. If they don't pass their exams, it isn't you who is going to live the results. It's them.

4. Wipe that destructive word 'always' right out of your vocabulary. Every time you are about to say 'You always ...' bite your tongue, even if it bleeds. It is only the present event that matters. How can anyone possibly expect or try to change if parents are determined to cast them into a mould of failure?

5. Use your head to make simple amendments to things which get on your nerves. If it's something as small and silly as putting the cap on the toothpaste, then get a new toothpaste that comes in an aerosol tin. If kids won't clear their junk, get a laundry basket, plonk all their things in it – dirty clothes, clean clothes, books, boots, records, anything – and leave it at the bottom of the stairs. Don't put them away.

6. If your child refuses to clean his or her room and lives in a pig sty, shut the door and leave it alone. Why fuss yourself? If it begins to smell, or seems like encouraging mice, you can order or organise a major clean up for health reasons. But frankly there are other more important issues at stake, not least your own peace of mind. The house won't collapse if one room is a mess but your peace of mind will be unnecessarily shattered if you try to butt your head against the brick wall of a teenager's obstinacy.

Ignore it. Save your energy for better things.

Covering Up (which is another way of saying **Lying**)

Now you know something about drugs and their effects, the manner of use and the consequences, you cannot plead ignorance, at least in the same degree. You may still not have smoked a joint or taken a fix but you know a bit more about it than when you started reading this book.

88

If you have reason to believe your child is obsessively gambling, compulsively drinking or becoming habituated to illicit drugs, trust your gut feeling. If any of these apply, then the teenager is suffering from an illness, the first and most prominent symptom of which is telling lies.

If you want to save your child's life, *don't go along with the lies.* There's no need to get into an argument, just make it quite clear you are aware that he or she is not telling the truth. At this stage there may not be anything else much that you can do about it, but it's a start.

The next symptom is trouble with either school, employer (if any) or the law. Or they start stealing from you. Here's where you have to begin exercising your real parent-power. The worst thing you can do for your youngster is to bail them out of trouble.

If stealing is the problem take action. The first few times it happens, chances are you persuade yourself you didn't really have that five pounds in your wallet or handbag anyway. That old silver clock of grandmother's is probably in a cupboard somewhere. In your heart you know the truth but it's the hardest thing in the world to admit your child is a thief.

This is where you begin to work. You have to tell your child you know what is going on. You have to set limits and make clear that this or that will happen if they do it again. What 'this or that' will be, must be something you know you can make stick. If you are going to expect a certain standard of behaviour, you have got to keep that standard yourself. If you say you will do something, you do it.

Maybe you'll fail the first few times. Don't worry, all parents do. It's incredibly hard to resist the blandishments, the endearing promises to reform, your own sheer fright for your youngster. Everyone fails a few times. But bit by bit, if you try to remember why you are being firm, you will gradually get the strength to do it.

The alternative is infinitely worse. Prison and suicide are common outcomes of addiction to gambling. Both of those, together with severe mental and physical damage are the consequences of addiction to alcohol or drugs.

So when you allow your youngster to face the magistrates, to be confronted with the law, to be expelled from school or college, when you allow him or her to experience the consequences of their own actions, you are giving them their right to learn by their own mistakes. Clearly they were not willing to learn by warnings. If you interfere, if you pay off their fines, intercede with the authorities, make promises on their behalf, how can they learn? You are depriving them of the privilege of growth.

As I have consistently emphasised, each case is different, every parent can only do what feels right. But the rightness is the rightness of your gut feeling, not a response to age-old sayings like, 'He's my flesh and blood, I'll see him through no matter what he does.' Those old saws simply do not work in the business of addiction. There's more at stake here than family honour, reputations or what the neighbours say. Addiction in any of these forms can lead to death, a very painful and degraded death at that.

Davina, a now-recovering heroin addict said, 'My parents kept covering up for me, getting me out of messes, paying off my debts. It wasn't till Daddy said he'd had enough, I was on my own, that the whole horror of my life became clear to me. I went into treatment, and I've been clean for three years now.'

David started using marijuana at thirteen. He quickly began experimenting with all kinds of other drugs. He left home at sixteen to live in squats and follow the addict life-style (though he called it the alternative society). Quite often he came home to 'crash out', get properly fed, have his bundle of squalid clothes put through the washing machine, borrow some cash from his mother (a single parent), then return to his druggy companions. His mother, unknowingly, was really providing a kind of hippy health-farm for him, getting him in shape for the next few weeks or months of self destruction. She believed she was 'keeping up a line of communication'. What can a mother do but take in her thin and shabby child, feed and water him, try to love him back to health and sanity? In fact she was in despair for two years until she began to learn to act on the principles this book is about.

90

One night the police came to the door. Did David live at this address? She acknowledged that it was his home but that he was away 'staying with friends'. Knowing the answer, she asked why the officers needed to know. 'He's being held on a drugs charge in X.' They gave her the number of a police station. She telephoned, found out that he was in a cell and was told that after the substance had been analysed, he would be released next morning following a routine appearance before the magistrates.

At two in the morning she had a call from one of the 'friends' – in fact a lad whom she knew to be a dealer. He begged her to ring the police and say that David would be living with her because without an address, he would probably be held on remand when charged. It could mean anything from three to twelve months in prison if had 'NFA' (No Fixed Abode) and hence could not be allowed bail.

Not quite believing it was her own voice, she heard herself saying 'No, I cannot tell the police that. It's a lie. He no longer really lives here'. The dealer pleaded, saying what a lovely guy David was. She answered clearly and firmly, 'I know that. It's because I love him I will not lie for him. Tell him I love him enough to let him take the consequences of his own actions.' She put the telephone down, and actually slept. In her heart she knew she had done the right thing, tough and terrible as it seemed.

In some amazing way (addict youngsters can be very persuasive) David was allowed out on his own cognizance. He went to stay with his dealer friend and did not even telephone her for about six weeks. She then told him she believed him to be ill and that she would do her best to get him into treatment. He put the telephone down on her.

But parent-power had begun to work. Not long afterwards, David started to clean up the squat he went to live in, but when the druggies kept coming back, he took a room in a 'straight' house – and then, to the family's amazement, got a real job. He's twenty two now and hasn't used a drug (except for a couple of brief and nasty relapses) for over two years.

Cheerfulness

No, I'm not joking. Your world has tumbled about your ears. Your once-beautiful child now a sad, unlovely wreck, your whole family is tense and miserable, facing all kinds of emotional or even real bankruptcy – and I'm talking about cheerfulness?

If you have been working on your own life, and taking your attention away from your sick child, you will find this a good deal easier. You will have things to think about that are not concerned with what the afflicted one is up to, or what they are going to do or what they might have been doing. You will be able, at least at intervals, to be thinking about your own life and what you are doing with it.

Secondly, you may have to start by acting 'as if'. This is a highly recommended way of making things happen. Start by uncracking the face. See what a smile feels like for a change. Gently smooth out your forehead, the edges beside your eyes, and with both hands, peacefully massage your cheeks upwards. Feels good, doesn't it? Now a smile?

When someone comes in, try it out for size. After weeks or months of frowns, disapproval or tears, it will probably come as quite a shock, not only to your erring youngster but even to the rest of the family, when you turn on a smile.

I cannot promise you a smile in return. But the more you practise 'as if' all was right, the more things are going to be. It may get worse – indeed, in many cases it *must* get worse before it gets better but it will have an effect.

Your addicted child will certainly be affected. Up till now, he or she has been not only unhappy and distressed, but has had the comfort (however peculiar it may sound) of knowing that you were distressed and unhappy too. Because all addiction produces emotional immaturity and dependence, the fact that mum and dad were worried, took away any urgent need to worry about themselves. But when the rest of the family starts being quite cheerful, getting along quite happily with their own lives and not agonising about the addict/alcoholic/gambler, some of the reality of his or her own situation comes home to roost. It's his or her problem, not yours, and only he or she can deal with it.

Another reason is equally cogent. The drug scene may not seem any too joyful to you but the 'straight' scene, i.e. home, is certainly not going to win any converts if everyone is going round with sad and sour faces and never a smile or laugh. You may not – yet – be able to get rid of the twist in your stomach every time you set eyes on your sick child, but for everyone's sake, put on a smile. It pays dividends. What's more, it comes easier with practice.

Courtesy

Grunts and sullen silences from uncouth teenagers do not exactly encourage one to behave as if at a Buckingham Palace tea party. On the other hand, there is no reason on earth why an unkempt teenager should dictate how an adult behaves.

Because a troublesome youth has no manners, does that mean *you* have to forget yours? Are you going to allow the brat to bring you down to his or her level? Unflagging courtesy is very undermining if your child is trying to get your back up. But do not confuse courtesy with grovelling. Good manners on your part does not mean that you allow your child to walk all over you. It is important to say 'please' and 'thank you' when requesting things to be done. It is not good manners to allow yourself to be rubbished.

Let us take an example. A plate of food is put before your son. He takes a forkful and pushes his plate away rudely, saying, 'Yah, I can't eat that muck.' What do you do?

1. Ask him what he'd like and offer to go and make it?
2. Point out that you've spent ages making it, because you thought he liked it and how were you to know he'd changed his taste?
3. Apologise because it wasn't as good as the last time?
4. Beg him to try a little more, he's so thin, he needs building up?

93

5. Tell him he'll sit there until he *does* eat it?
6. Give him a cuff over the head and tell him to get on with it?
7. Order him to leave and stay in his room for the rest of the night?
8. Tell him not to speak to you/his mother like that?
9. Tell him pleasantly to take his plate to the kitchen, and that he may leave the table?
10. Say, 'What a shame. Better have some bread and cheese then.'

The first four make you a walkover or a whiner. The next three (5,6 & 7) are bullying dead-ends leading straight into a row. You could paraphrase it into 'taking a mule to the table but not being able to make him eat'. Number 8 may have some value, depending on who says it and in what tone of voice. Only you can know whether it is likely to work or whether it has been said so often it's a bore. But certainly 9 and 10 are the most effective responses. You are not making a mountain out of a molehill. You aren't letting him wind the family up. His attempt to cause trouble falls on stony ground. Round one to the parents. Every time a row is sidestepped without anyone losing face, you're winning.

On the other hand it is *not* polite to make rude remarks about their new clothing or taste in music. It's legitimate to expect music to be played at a decibel level that won't interfere with your convenience. It is *not* polite to make disparaging remarks about the music itself. Even if s/he snarls at your taste in music, *their* bad manners do not mean you lose *yours*.

If you're saddled with a punk try to think positively about it. This really is a phase. Nobody stays a punk forever. All the hours (and money) spent in creating an amazing colourful image with those perfect, symmetrical spikes down the head! What artistry! Underneath that brilliant, meticulous creation is probably a very frightened, very lost, spotty boy or girl, with no sense of direction, no job prospects, and no sense of future.

It may seem to you to be a dreadful waste of time and money but it helps if you think of them as an actor about to walk out on a stage. That the stage is the street corner where they'll only

94

meet yet more punks, equally bedecked, is neither here nor there. It is at least an act of creation, no more dangerous in itself than a master chef who spends hours making fantastic confections designed to be eaten at the next banquet.

Everyone wants to do something well. Most punks would probably prefer to be recognised because they had actually *done* something – climbed Everest, walked on the moon, got to the top of the charts – but to date they haven't. The only available recognition for a punk is to turn heads in the street. Even disapproval is better than anonymity.

So, don't cut a punk down to size. Try (however hard) to admire the artistry. That rose bed you put so much time into, is that any more valuable than your own child? That they put the effort into making a different self-image is not such a far cry from your rosebed. Left to itself, the garden would soon run to weeds and nettles. Nature, without human help, makes a lousy gardener. So be civil to your punk. It costs nothing and it can only make him or her feel better to get a little admiration from the family – of all people!

The Big H

No, it's not heroin, it's honesty. And if you have read this far, you will have noticed that honesty is what it is all about.

We have seen that dishonesty is the immediate and most evident symptom of trouble when addiction or dependence is in question. For that reason, health and recovery begins and grows with honesty.

Honesty comes in all sizes. It comes in the obvious ways – like paying the bills and giving value for money. It means being honest at work, at home and in business.

But it also means being honest with yourself, and about yourself.

Honesty demands great courage. It means putting yourself on the line. It often means you have to take risks. You have to risk your child's displeasure, even the fear that he or she may love you less. In practice, such a thing never happens. When you pull your two year old child away from a dangerous dog that it wants to pat, you don't lose the child's love, although it may beat you and wail heartbrokenly. Likewise when you refuse to accept lies from your troubled teenager, you may get a mouthful (in the short term) but you gain respect in the long run. Honesty means doing what you know, in your gut, to be right.

Honesty involves taking a good long look at yourself and accepting that you are often less than perfect. It means also admitting that you have a whole lot of good in you. You are kind? Compassionate? Warm hearted? A good friend? You have talent? You're a hard worker? You're a good father? Mother? Employer? Employee? You want the best for your family. You have worked hard for it. You are *not* inadequate. You have never wanted to harm anyone and you have not failed, though you may have sometimes been mistaken.

Honesty requires that you recognise and acknowledge your real feelings. If right this minute you are angry with your child (or your partner or anyone else for that matter) accept that this is how you feel, just for today. Accept the fact of your feelings. There is simply no point in saying to yourself 'I ought to feel love for …' when you damned well don't. But honesty demands that you look a bit further and try to find out what it is in yourself that has sparked off this anger. Is it guilt? Pride? Something in yourself that you recognise in the other person?

It has been said that when I criticise someone for something they have done, it is because I too have either done it, am doing it or want to do it. If I criticise someone for talking all the time, you can be sure that that is one of my own worst failings.

'What you are shouts so loudly that I cannot hear what you say,' says the sage. Honesty demands that we behave according to the words which come out of our mouths.

It is simply no good for a father who staggers into the house after nights at the pub to start sounding off at his druggy son. OK, the drugs may be illegal but the intoxication is common to both. Honesty demands that we clean up our own act. Hypocrisy is dishonesty in refined form.

Honesty requires that we look at our reasons for doing things. If I like a tidy house, then I tidy it. I do *not* tidy it for someone else. I tidy it because I like it that way. My children may be entirely happy in a disorderly house. I can limit their disorder to their own spaces, I can take steps to ensure that my spaces are not invaded by their mess. But I cannot with honesty tell them I keep the place tidy 'for them'.

Likewise, if I choose to spend long hours at work (or the golf club) rather than go home to tedious chores like mowing the lawn or taking my children to the park I stop kidding everyone, in particular myself, that it's all about 'furthering my career prospects' or 'keeping up our standard of living'. The practice of honesty may be costly, but the pay-off is concerned not so much with my standard of living but, more importantly, with the quality of life.

Being honest means I stop playing the martyr. Martyrs are in the business of getting power through pity. Parent-power is another bag altogether. Parent-power grows out of honesty, not out of self-pity.

Honesty means I stop bullying. A bullying father who uses his weight and size to intimidate his youngster has already lost the battle. Whether his weapons are words or fists, he admits with every blow the poverty of his resources. The bully hurts inside and getting the courage to face that pain is the toughest job a bully can do. It means admitting that your pride is hurt, that you feel impotent, that the situation is out of control, that you are lost and frightened and bewildered. But out of these admissions can come the strength to accept that you *can* change yourself, a day at a time, and help to change the whole situation.

Honesty expects that we stop being so darned smug. When I say to my child, 'In my day I had to rise at dawn, work for sixteen hours, eat bread and dripping ...' and so on and so on, what I'm really saying is, 'Look at me now, aren't I marvellous?' Well, to the prejudiced eye of my child I am probably very far from marvellous. To be frank, I'm probably a great big smug pain in the neck. I can stop pretending that the sun shines out of me, because it just doesn't. I can think before I talk. When my child answers, 'but it was different in your day,' that child is saying no less than the truth.

In my day, and in yours, teenagers were probably not even invented. One was a child, then one was an 'in-between' or 'at the difficult age' and of no possible consequence in the scheme of things.

Things *are* different now. Teenagers are a commercial resource. They are the big buyers of cosmetics and music, of clothes and drink and drugs. They're fodder not only for commerce but also for the caring industries: for the youth workers, the researchers, the social workers, and the hordes of civil servants who are paid to plan how they occupy their time. Where would all these industries be without the raw material of teenagers? That's a far cry from the way it was when we were spotty sixteen year olds.

Honesty gets you everywhere. It can sometimes be painful, but the rewards are unexpectedly great. In honesty rests the key to your recovery. Through honesty you regain your self-esteem, your self-confidence and your self-respect. In honesty lies the secret of parent-power at its most potent.

FOUR

WHERE THE HELP IS

Most young alcoholics (provided they are not cross-addicted) will not need medical treatment for withdrawal. For gamblers, there is no physical withdrawal to contend with. Drug addicts, depending on the substances they have been using may need medical help in withdrawing.

In the general way it is possible to come off anything, if just for a day. The major problem with addiction is not stopping, but *staying stopped*. Unless your youngster is going to stay confined to the house when they kick the habit, they are going to find it quite rough out there. They need not only new friends, but a new way to live, happily and contentedly, without the ups and downs, the highs and lows that are part and parcel of addiction. If the addict, alcoholic or gambler doesn't change their attitudes, behaviour and actions, they will inevitably go back to addiction in one or other of its shapes. Unless life without a drink, pill, fix or 'machine' becomes good, inevitably they will turn again to the drink, pill, fix or amusement arcade.

Many of them got into the scene through 'friends'. The easy way to get out of it is also through friends, but friends who have been through the pain and anguish, the fear and despair of addiction, who have learnt (and are still learning) new ways to stay straight, clean, sober and happy today.

Walk into any AA meeting and you will find yourself among a complete cross-section of your neighbourhood. There'll be people of all ages, from all walks of life, classes and back-grounds. Just as the illness of alcoholism is no respecter of persons, you might find the person sitting next to you is a docker or a doctor, an air-stewardess or a priest, an unemployed labourer or a pregnant mum. What they do is not important. How they are, is. And how they are is sober. They are there for the sole reason that AA enables them to get and to stay sober, a day at a time.

Narcotics Anonymous, going strong in the US, is only recently arrived in the UK and there are not very many meetings, but practically all the members are young. Any two recovering addicts can easily find out how to start meeting to help themselves and others to recover.

Gamblers Anonymous have only recently become aware of the need for young people's groups – but addicts of all kinds know that the illness does not make distinctions of age, sex, colour, race or creed.

For problem drinkers: *Alcoholics Anonymous*
                          Telephone number can be found
                          in your local directory.

For problem gamblers: *Gamblers Anonymous*
                          Find telephone number in local
                          directory.

For problems with drugs: *Narcotics Anonymous*
                          PO Box 246,
                          London SW10
                          Telephone: (01) 351 6794